Inside Syria - A Physician's Memoir by Tarif Bakdash, MD, is authentic and brave and from the heart.

—Stephen Fife author of *The 13th Boy* and
Dreaming in the Maze of Love-Grief-Madness

Watching news footage of Syrian refugees trekking through Europe, I've wished I had a Syrian friend to tell me what's going on. Reading Tarif Bakdash's *Inside Syria - A Physician's Memoir*, I have found that friend. Tarif Bakdash is a Syrian-American MD who practices and teaches at a medical college in Wisconsin.

Dr Bakdash's memoir tells the story of two journeys. The physical journey dominates the book. It starts with a boyhood in war-scarred Syria where international conflict is a fact of life. In 1988, it follows Tarif to the United States where for 14 years he pursues medical studies and a career that combines practice and teaching at American hospitals.

Although he becomes an American, Tarif's heart never really leaves Syria. In 2002, after the passing of the dictator-tyrant Hafez al-Assad, he returns to Damascus, hoping to help build a different kind of country. Blocked at every turn, he comes back to the US in 2010 just before the government crackdown on peaceful protest which gave rise to the chaos now engulfing Syria.

Dr Bakdash's second journey is a spiritual one. His study of Sufiism, undertaken in the US, leads him from "the Quran of legalism" into "the Quran of mercy," envisioning a spiritual family that includes all men and women. He calls his book "my *jihad* on behalf of the Quran of peace."

Hundreds of thousands of migrants are bringing Syria and the Quran to the West. It behooves Westerners to learn about this society. Reading *Inside Syria - A Physician's Memoir*, is an excellent place to start. Highly recommended.

—Frederic Hunter author of *A Year in the Jungle* and
The Girl Ran Away

Dr Bakdash is a pediatric neurologist who worked with Syrian children in our clinic at the Za'atari Refugee Camp in Jordan. He used his education, skills, and knowledge to help young Syrians who had lost everything—everything, that is, except hope. His warmth, drive, dedication, and humble manner were exceptional. He put a smile on every face.

—Dr MK Hamza
  Syrian American Medical Society
  Lamar University

At the time I was a young Mom raising my two-year-old son when he was diagnosed with a significant disorder. I was afraid of what was to come and felt alone in this journey. This is how I met Dr Bakdash and from that day, my life was blessed with a new friend. Sometimes in this world we get the chance to meet great people that change our lives. Dr Bakdash started a non-profit organization named KODI, to help parents of children that had been affected by neurological disorders and diseases. I was asked to be a board member of this group and help other families that were going through similar situations as mine. The kindness, support and love Tarif showed to these families has made a tremendous impact on their lives as well as mine.

—Brynn
  Grand Junction, Colorado

In 2015, Dr Bakdash received the Standing Ovation Award from the Children's Hospital of Wisconsin.

When my daughter started experiencing symptoms that no one could explain, I went to our local hospital where I met Dr Bakdash. He presented himself with a gentle handshake as though he was just an ordinary man. Still, I sensed that he was a man of great knowledge. Dr Bakdash spoke with amazing supportive eloquence. Surrounding him was an aura of peace and calmness. My daughter's anxiety about the visit melted.

Dr Bakdash spent time with us to answer *all* of our questions. He ensured that, before we left his office, we were comfortable with what he believed was going on and what was going to happen next. His willingness to connect with us on a personal level made us feel as though we were part of a family and that he truly deeply cared about us as people.

—Andrea
East Troy, Wisconsin

In a world that lacks compassion you will find that Dr Bakdash is a rare treasure that goes above and beyond for all with a compassionate and warm heart. His selfless acts for humanity inspire me to be a better person. Not only did I find a great doctor for my child but a true friend as well.

—Alicia
Milwaukee

To God
To the Scientific and Merciful Islam
To My Fellow Americans and Syrians
To My Parents and Family
To Humanity

Inside Syria —
A Physician's Memoir

Inside Syria —
A Physician's Memoir

My Life as a Child, a Student, and an MD in an Era of War

Tarif Bakdash, MD
WD Blackmon

 Cune

Inside Syria—A Physician's Memoir:
My Life as a Child, a Student, and an MD in an Era of War
by Tarif Bakdash, MD and WD Blackmon
© 2016 Tarif Bakdash and WD Blackmon
Cune Press, Seattle 2016 First Edition 2 4 6 8 9 7 5 3

Hardback	ISBN 9781614571643	$24.95
Kindle (pre-publication excerpt)	ISBN 9781614571667	$ .99
Kindle	ISBN 9781614571674	$ 9.99

Names: Bakdash, Tarif, author. | Blackmon, W. D., transcriber. | Ferzat,
Ali., illustrator.
Title: Inside Syria--a physician's memoir : my life as a child, a student &
an MD in an era of war / by Tarif Bakdash, as told to W.D. Blackmon ;
illustrator Ali Ferzat.
Description: Seattle : Cune Press, [2016] | Includes bibliographical
references.
Identifiers: LCCN 2015027033| ISBN 9781614571643 (hardback) | ISBN
9781614571650 (paperback) | ISBN 9781614571667 (eBook) | ISBN
9781614571674 (Kindle)
Subjects: LCSH: Bakdash, Tarif. | Physicians--United States--Biography. |
Assad, Bashar, 1965- | Medicine--Practice--Syria. | Medical care--Corrupt
practices--Syria. | Medicine--Practice--United States. | Syria--Politics
and government--2000- | Syria--Politics and government--1971-2000.
Classification: LCC R722.32.B35 A3 2015 | DDC 610.95691--dc23
LC record available at http://lccn.loc.gov/2015027033

Cover photo © 2016 Tarif Bakdash (Za'atari refugee camp in Jordan, 2015)
Political cartoons: © 2016 Ali Ferzat (also Farzat or Firzat) from *A Pen of Damascus Steel*
and *The Arab-American Handbook* (Cune Press).

Other Books in the Syria Crossroads Series from Cune Press:

East of the Grand Umayyad	Sami Moubayed
The Plain of Dead Cities	Bruce McLaren
Steel & Silk	Sami Moubayed
Syria - A Decade of Lost Chances	Carsten Wieland
The Road from Damascus	Scott C. Davis
A Pen of Damascus Steel	Ali Ferzat

Coming Soon:

Leaving Syria	Bassam S. Rifai
Art in Exile	Natasha Hamarneh Hall
Gate of Peace, Gate of Wind	Patrick Hilsman
Quwatli	Sami Moubayed

Cune Press: www.cunepress.com | www.cunepress.net
Cune Press is a project of the Salaam Cultural Museum.
Salaam delivers aid to Syrian refugees:
www.salaamculturalmuseum.org | www.scmmedicalmissions.org

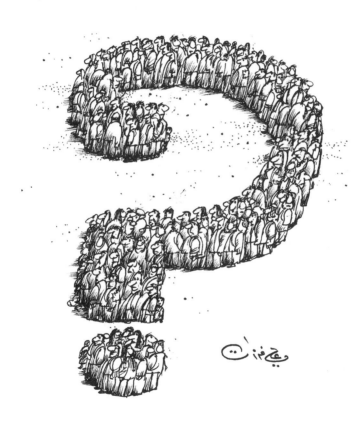

Contents

Illustrations by Ali Ferzat

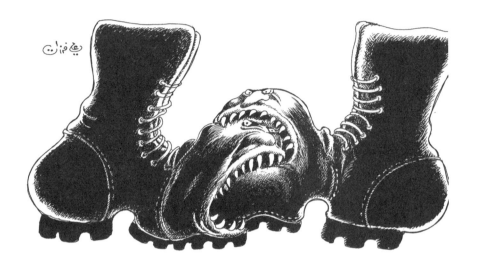

My Life in an Era of War

The following timeline sketches my life and the military conflicts that provided the backdrop to everyday events in my world.

1948   Arab-Israeli War (Palestinians term this the *Nakba*. Many Palestinian families displaced in 1948 are still living in refugee camps)

1965   Tarif was born in Damascus. His father worked in a bank, and the family lived in the upscale Malki neighborhood

1967   Six-Day War with Israel, resulted in the loss of the Golan

1970   Black September: Syrians fought in Jordan to protect Palestinians
        Tarif lived in Morroco for one year

1971   Tarif began a two-year stay in Beirut

1973   Yom Kippur War: Syria and Egypt attacked Israel to recover land lost in 1967

1976   The Lebanese Civil War began

1979   The Muslim Brotherhood uprising in Syria began

1980   Tarif's schoolmates were arrested on suspicion of supporting the Muslim Brotherhood

1982   With the Hama massacre, the Muslim Brotherhood was defeated

1985   Tarif and his father visited his uncle in Minnesota for three weeks and Tarif received a green card

1988   Tarif completed his medical studies and "escaped" to Jordan, then traveled to the US

1990   The Lebanese Civil War ended

2002   Tarif returned to Syria at age thirty-seven to teach at the University of Damascus and to engage in private practice

2007   Tarif begins working with AAMAL, the first lady's charity for the disabled

2009   Tarif met his future wife in Damascus (married in 2012)
        Tarif was named the Secretary General for the Disabled in Syria

2010   Tarif left Syria and returned to the US

2011   Syrian Civil War began

2015   In April, Tarif returned to the Middle East for eight days to treat Syrian refugees at the Za'atari refugee camp in Jordan

Note to the Reader

I have heard the Messenger of God [peace be upon him] say: "If any of you see something wrong he must try and change it with his hand, and if he is unable then with his tongue, and if he is unable then with his heart . . ."

—Hadith, Abu Sa'eed al-Khudree

"Tarif, why? Why are you doing this?" It's my brother Samer asking these questions. And, older by two years, he has a right to ask.

"What right do you have to speak against Assad?" He looked at me, then continued. "You don't live in Syria anymore. You left. I stayed. What do you gain by writing against the regime? How does it help you, your family, my family, our friends—the ones who stayed? You—you're not Syrian anymore."

He had a point. I did leave.

I had left for America once before, back in 1988, disgusted by the corruption and waste and hypocrisy and incompetency and sheer indecency of the Ba'athist regime. And I stayed in America for fourteen years, establishing myself as a practitioner and a teacher of pediatric neurology. Ironically, it was the installation of Bashar al-Assad as President that led me back to Syria. With the death of Bashar's father, Hafez, hope rose in me that Syria could grow beyond Ba'athism. In 2002, with the promise of new leadership, I was eager to return and to help, in whatever way I could, to improve the Syrian health care system.

The Assad family took personal interest in my efforts. Bashar himself arranged for my teaching appointment at the Damascus University Medical School and, several years later, his wife and Syrian First Lady, Asma al-Assad, secured my appointment as Director of Services for AAMAL, Asma's "signature" charity for the disabled in Syria. In 2009, I received a second appointment from Bashar himself, this time as the first Secretary General for the Disabled in Syria. With each new appointment, I tried—hard, in fact—to improve physician-training and health services generally, and for the disabled specifically. And I failed. So I left Syria a second time—for good, just five years ago.

In 2010, I came back to America with my mother, Nawal, and my father,

Fouad. I have an aunt and some cousins living in Jordan and Syria still, but, of my immediate family, only Samer remains in Damascus, he with his wife, Sereen, and their two children. He manages an insurance company—a rather chancy business in Syria today—*and keeps praying for the war to stop.*

"And have you forgotten?" was my response. "Have you forgotten the violence, the lies, the indignities of the past forty years?" Samer was born in 1963, I in 1965. Hafez al-Assad came to power in 1971 and ruled until his death in 2000, when he was succeeded by his second son, Bashar. So Samer and I grew up together in the same household in the same world under Assad. Samer knew very well what I was talking about.

"Tarif . . . brother," he said, stammering out a half-hearted self-defense. "What's the alternative? ISIS? Really? All I know is that I have to go back to Damascus. And if you write this book, you can never go back—never."

It might seem strange, but that thought had not really "sunk in" until Samer spoke it aloud for me. At the time of this conversation, I was already half-way through the writing of this present book. He had just flown in to Springfield, Missouri (where I'd been living with my wife, mother, and father), and I had just picked him up at the airport. This was supposed to be a happy reunion of family, but it wasn't starting out happily. I would have expected him to be gazing out of the car window in enjoyment of a fine spring day in the Ozarks region of Southwest Missouri, whose lush countryside contrasts so starkly with dusty Damascus. But, throughout our car-ride conversation, he looked down, staring into his lap. I don't know what I would have seen, had he let me look into his eyes.

"You're right," I replied. "I can't go back—that is, back to living the lies of Assad's Syria."

"Just think about what you're doing," he said. And, with that, I let him have the last word.

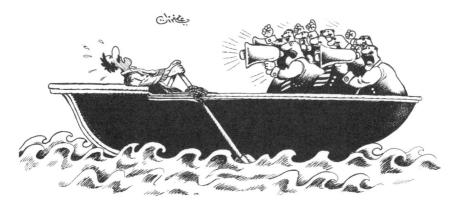

Springfield is a mid-sized Midwest town of about 150,000 that has just about everything one would expect from a mid-sized town in the American Midwest. It is sprawling and suburban and constantly expanding its boundaries—which is not all that difficult, given the expanses of land between Midwest towns. I'm told that its economy was once driven by manufacturing and the railroad. Now, its service-driven economy is dominated by health care and higher education (in effect, by hospitals and colleges). It's expansion within the former that brought me here. I worked in the "Mercy System," with its sprawling, multi-block medical campus just south of Sunshine Street (at one time the southernmost edge of town). St John's, as it was once called, was Springfield's first hospital, founded in 1891 by the Sisters of Mercy, a Catholic order of nuns who came south from St Louis. Apparently the largely Protestant townspeople didn't like the idea of being saved by Roman Catholics, so the Baptist Hospital opened its midtown doors in 1904 while the Methodist-affiliated Burge Deaconess Hospital opened in 1905 on the town's north side.[1] Now called the "Cox Health System," the old Burge Deaconess remains Mercy's main competitor, with Cox Medical Center South sitting just a few miles down the road, on a stretch of National Avenue known as Springfield's "medical mile."

From that last paragraph, one might get the impression that Springfield has a history of religious prejudice. Be that as it may, Springfieldians today work actively to heal the wounds that have marked its history. As I shall note throughout this memoir, I have never personally met with prejudice against my Muslim faith. With quizzical looks, yes, but with suspicious looks, no—not in Springfield.

After that first foray with Samer, we drove in silence. I wanted to break the ice and say something about the town we were heading toward, but all I could think to do was point out a few obvious landmarks. Samer glanced at each and nodded.

Samer's Springfield trip was too brief, though it became tense at times when conversation turned to politics in the Middle East. When I drove him back to the airport for his flight home, his words sounded like a broken record. "Just think about what you're doing."

I kissed him farewell.

* * *

When I began writing this memoir, I was living in Springfield, working as a pediatric neurologist in a clinic tied to Mercy Hospital. I was also member of the hospital's ethics committee—which at first surprised me, since Mercy remains affiliated with the Catholic Church and I'm a devout Muslim. More specifically, I am a Sufi-inspired Muslim who believes, with all his heart, that the Quran is a book of peace and that the true message of the Quran has been grossly, grotesquely, sinfully, indeed blasphemously distorted by Islamist radicals.

My wife, Remaz, is a Palestinian whom I met in Syria. She has just lately obtained her green card and is busy improving her English. There's some irony in her as-yet halting English, since her lilting Arab voice was heard regularly on Arabesque FM 102.3, a radio station in Damascus. In fact, she was working for Rotana TV—part of the Arab world's largest entertainment group, owned by Saudi Prince Al-Waleed bin Talal—before our marriage and migration to the States. When world celebrities or musicians visited Damascus, Rotana sent her to interview them.

Few Damascenes will remember the public-service radio and television interviews that I gave during my years at AAMAL, but many will remember Remaz. She still has her fans, in fact. And why shouldn't she? She's charming, engaging, and empathetic. Remaz's story, and the story of her family, is a book in itself. Though her passport declares her Syrian citizenship, her Palestinian grandparents fled from Israeli-occupied Golan, making her a third-generation refugee. And though she achieved minor fame in Syrian radio and entertainment television, she left it all behind when the bombs started falling.

Her brother Hassan Sahtout, who is a pediatric surgeon, has also managed to flee with his wife and three children, though their path was more circuitous and dangerous. Travelling from Syria to Egypt and then Libya, he knew that their only chance for freedom lay in asylum in Europe. So, leaving his wife and children behind, he joined several male friends in a rubber dinghy. For 47 hours, they fought the Mediterranean Sea and winds to reach the Italian shore. From Italy, he boarded a plane for Sweden, where he applied for asylum for his family. This was in 2013. He lives safely and happily in Sweden now, with his wife and children.

My Syrian-born father, Fouad, is eighty-four years old. To me, his baldness shows off the perfect oval of his face, which sits atop his compact five foot nine inch frame. Though slowing physically, he's sharp as a tack mentally and a congenial companion to my mother, Nawal. Over the years, his native kindness and gentility have deepened, making him the family's peacekeeper. He's a good listener and always thinks before he speaks, which ensures the soundness of his advice. I am honored to call him my father, my confidant, and my friend.

A retired banker and accountant, Fouad's fortunes rose and fell with each change of regime. As the reader might guess, I'm relieved that he has joined me here in the States.

My Jordanian-born mother, Nawal, is seventy-five going on sixty, as they say in Springfield—despite injuries that she's suffered over the years. Her five foot four inch frame compels her to look up to most people, but her personality projects as much, much bigger. Strong-willed and opinionated, she's the family matriarch, indeed. As I look upon her, the years have brought little change. She wears her hair the same way that she did in her thirties and she speaks in the same way, thinks in the same way—and, I suppose, feels in the same way. Despite her streak of independence—she was a successful entrepreneur-businesswoman in a male-dominated Arab world—no one in her family has ever doubted her fierce loyalty or the strength of her love.

Much of Nawal's story is interwoven with mine, so I'll not give details here. All I'll note is that she has made great sacrifices on our family's behalf, and I honor her for those sacrifices. I love my mother dearly and I'm glad that she's here in the States living with her husband, my wife, and me.

I've already written some about my older brother, Samer. Standing six feet four inches tall, he's always topped me by a few inches (and a few pounds). Still, he's his father's son, with the same oval of a face and the same pattern baldness. He graduated from Damascus University with a degree in electrical engineering, but he's a "people person" and the most affable of our little family, so it made sense that he would go on to take coursework in business.

It's not just his business connections but his friendships that have kept him in Damascus. Since his Springfield visit, however, the war has come closer to his doorstep. A bomb fell in the lot just behind his office, shattering glass. While he was driving, bombs were dropping on the street behind him—literally. And he has fewer friends now, for some have fled while some have been lost to violence.

I've already noted Samer's response to my writing of this memoir. My wife, I should add, supports me in the writing. My parents, like my brother, do not.

"As a mother, I beg you. Do not let my son do this." Thus began a conversation that was recounted to me by a friend—a colleague of my co-author—who offered help in editing this book. He had arranged for studio portraits and, while I was having my photo taken, Nawal took my friend aside and began working her persuasion.

"Here, let me show you photos of my family." She got out her iPhone and called up her electronic photo album. There were pictures of Fouad in middle

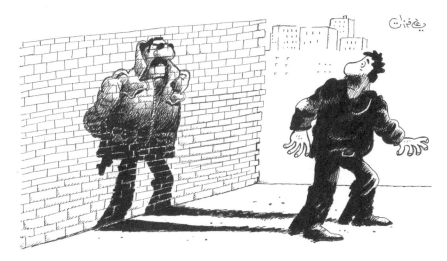

age, of me as a child, of Samer more recently with his wife and children.

The reader needs to understand that our little family lived near the Assad family's Damascus neighborhood. That I attended medical school with Bashar al-Assad. And that I worked for three years with the Syrian President's wife, Asma al-Assad, to develop nonprofit initiatives aiding people with disabilities. For now, that's all I'll write on these topics. But all that should explain why my mother would corner my friend in this way.

"I want to be able to go back home," my mother continued. "I have family in Damascus. If Tarif writes this book, how can I go back? How can he go back? He will be killed. Please, as a mother, I beg you. Stop him from doing this." And my friend, following his conscience, promised to do his best. He could not stop me, but he could advise me and warn me.

That weekend after the photo-shoot, the three of us—my friend, my co-author, and I—met at the local Barnes & Noble over coffee. My friend had convened the meeting, intending to carry out his promise.

"Look me in the eye, Tarif," my friend said, leaning in toward me. "Look me in the eye and tell me that no one will get hurt from your writing."

"I can't," was my simple, honest response. Of course I said more. "As a Muslim, a humanitarian, and an ethicist, I must be true to my calling," I told them. "The truth is worth the risk. One can't justify evil by declaring someone or something else 'more evil.' My aim isn't simply to expose Ba'athism or call Bashar al-Assad to justice. My aim, rather, is to express the true Islam, which stands for peace—not war."

"And I owe this book," I said at last, "to all moderate, peace-loving Muslims, who find their faith disfigured by radicalism. I owe it to those many

Americans who have not heard of the Quran of peace and who find only fear and suspicion and confusion in Islam. And I owe it to God. If you wish, you can call this book my jihad on behalf of the Quran of peace."

"And the timing is right, besides," my co-author added.

Well, my friend is a devout Christian and for every Quranic verse that I can quote he's quick to find a Bible equivalent.

"Blessed are the feet of them that preach the gospel of peace," he said.

"Yes," I said, "and the Muslim greeting, *salam* or *salam alaykum*, means 'peace.' The word Islam itself derives from *salam*—from 'peace.'"

"But . . . think hard about what you're doing," he rejoined, and then sighed. "Consider yourself warned."

"All I can do," I replied, "is tell the truth without anger, avoid caricature and name-calling, confess my own frailties, and trust in God."

With that, my friend let me have the last word. Our conversation turned to other topics.

* * *

I did take some lessons from the above conversations. Though I'm writing in a land where free speech is guaranteed, I'm sensitive to the hazards of writing of a regime where political enemies—and the friends and relatives of enemies—suffer retribution. For the sake of friends and relatives, I've omitted or changed some names. After all, I've left but many have stayed behind in Ba'athist Syria, where the best protection is often silence. Power demands genuflection. I do not blame those who make a show of obedience and support to the regime of Bashar al-Assad, since they still have to live their lives as best they can—and I do not want my stories to make it harder for them.

I say "stories," since there are several narratives interwoven through the chapters that follow.

The first narrative presents a Syrian-born physician's version of events from the formation of "Black September" in 1970 through the current Syrian crisis. I write as an eye-witness and, occasionally, as a minor participant in Syrian affairs. I write "minor participant," since my work on behalf of the disabled would barely register as a "blip" on the Assad regime's radar screen. But to me, of course, my work back then mattered, and I know of no other Syrian who has written with as much intimacy of detail regarding the state of medicine (and of medical training) in my native country. With my immigration to America in 2010, the first installment of this memoir comes to an end.

My chapter-postscript or "coda" focuses on Syrian affairs after March 2011, when the nationwide protests—peaceful protests, mind you—began in earnest. Repressed by the Ba'athists, these grew into the civil war still raging today. Of these more recent events, I write not as an eye-witness but as a bystander—not as a Syrian living in Damascus but as a Syrian-American who must gather his information second-hand through email and cellphone and, more chancy, through the filtered, cropped, distorted, even censored Internet and television news. (In this respect, I'm as interested in the Western media's *representations* of Syria as much as in the events themselves.)

After months of hand-wringing indecision, it was in September 2014 that the US began taking the Syrian-Iraqi ISIS threat seriously and air strikes began—not just in Iraq, but in Syria. American missiles have fallen on Syrian soil. For good or ill, this intervention has shifted the dynamics of the Syrian crisis. What Assad's atrocities against his own people could not do, mass executions by the so-called Islamic State have at last accomplished. They have gotten the attention of the US and other Western powers, who now acknowledge that the terror emanating from ISIS cannot be quarantined.

The Russian Federation, in contrast, stands in continued support of the Assad regime. Russian air strikes from their base in Latakia have primarily targeted opponents of Assad, although the recent downing of a Russian airliner over the Sinai Peninsula has moved the Russians to target ISIS as well. In regard to Russian support for Syria, little has changed from the old Soviet Union. Russia is still propping up the Syrian government and teaching Ba'athists the fine art of manipulating a nation's people.

As a physician, I hate to politicize disease, even metaphorically. But recent outbreaks of Ebola (for which physicians have scrambled to find a cure) and MERS cannot be contained in our current, "small world" globalism. As people travel, their infections travel with them—and so Africa's Ebola crisis becomes the world's crisis. Similarly with ISIS and other radicalized cults of terror. As with Ebola, one can say that there is as yet "no known cure" or clear solution to the sectarian violence spreading throughout the Middle East and North Africa.

Earlier in September, before the bombing began, President Barak Obama admitted that his administration had yet to formulate a clear policy against ISIS. At least he was honest in admitting that the US, like other Western nations, possessed "no known cure" for this fast-spreading political disease. But, returning to the language of medicine, let me note that ISIS is not the original "infection" that has plagued Syria and Iraq for so long. Rather, the Islamic State is a co-infection now raging within the body-politic of two nations whose chronic illness has come from Ba'athism. And, as a physician, I know that health requires the curing of both—that is, of both the original infection and the co-infections developing thereafter.

I'm not so Quixotic as to think that I have found an easy cure, but I do believe that a long-term, lasting solution to Islamic radicalism will need to come from within the body of Islam itself. It will require a restoration of the true meaning of jihad and a reeducation of Islamic youth, both today and in the future. The "new curriculum," if I may call it such, will include coursework in humanitarian ethics, in democracy, in social justice, in equality, in economic opportunity, and in that truer understanding of Islam which I've taken to call "the Quran of peace." (There is another enlightened approach, which I call "the Quran of science." Perhaps as a sequel to this present memoir, I hope to write about it.)

When I say that it's possible for a Muslim to throw off prejudices and old hatreds and to experience a purification of the heart, I can point to a personal example: my own. For I was raised in a world of religious prejudice against Jews and, truth to tell, my family did suffer at the hands of Israelis. When I lived and studied in Syria, I did not know the Quran of peace. In fact, I'd say now that I didn't know the Quran, the *true* Quran, at all. Beyond fasting during Ramadan, my immediate family was not fastidiously observant. It's somewhat ironic to note, but I did not know the Quran of peace until I left Syria and came to study and practice medicine in America.

In America, literally for the first time in my life, I had unlimited, uncensored access to books and experienced genuine freedom of thought. I read—no, I devoured—books on philosophy, on ethics, and on Islam. In America, I actually *studied* Islam. And it was in America that I had my first, fateful confrontation with Sufism. I have come to the understanding that Sufism—the inner heart of Islam—offers the only sure antidote to Islamic radicalism and its distorted versions of the Quran.

The Sufi recognizes three levels of meaning in the Quran. Most people who call themselves Muslims practice (more or less) the first level, which is public and is duty-based and includes bearing witness that God is the only God and Mohammed is the prophet of God (along the line of all other prophets, including Jesus, Moses, and Abraham, peace be upon them), praying five times a day, paying Zakat (2.5% of one's annual income to help the poor), fasting during Ramadan for thirty days per year, and, finally, going on a Hajj once in a lifetime, if capable. The second level, labeled Iman (to believe), means believing in God, His angels, and His books (the Bible, the Torah, Quran, etc.), which means that any Muslim, by definition, is also a Christian and a Jew. It also means believing in doomsday and in a faith that comes from God. The third level, Ishan (beautification), means to worship God as if you see him, for, if you don't, he does see you. This will lead to beautifying your actions.

The first level is legalistic—pertaining to the observances of prayers and other rites and duties as outlined in the Quran, Hadith, and Sharia law. The second level is moral—when one lives in charity and justice towards others regardless of their faith or economic or social status. Some Muslims—though not enough—do practice the fullness of charity and justice as these are described in the Quran and Hadith. I write, "the fullness of charity and justice," since there are many in the Muslim world who do act charitably and justly to some—typically, to those of their own sect—but not to all. And by "all," I don't mean "to all Muslims," but rather "to all people." For the Quran of peace, as I've come to understand it, applies to all of God's children regardless of faith.

Fewer still reach the third level of meaning, which is internal and experiential—when we feel God's presence in our hearts and know, not just believe, but *know*, His mercy and loving kindness. And when we know His mercy and loving kindness and feel His constant presence in our hearts, we become human vessels and messengers of that same divine mercy and loving kindness. Prejudice, injustice, lack of forgiveness, indifference to others' suffering. These are the effects of a hardened, uncharitable heart that does not feel God's continual presence within. But when one feels that divine presence and acknowledges it and resolves to live within its pattern—that is, by performing acts of mercy and loving kindness—then prejudice, injustice, lack of forgiveness, and indifference melt away.

This third level inspires one to live morally, prayerfully, and in accordance with the law. How could it be otherwise, since acts of immorality and injustice cloud the presence of God within?—And who would deliberately cloud that presence which gives such bliss, such hope, such meaning to life?

In professing this truer understanding, I'm proud to declare myself a fan of Seyyed Hossein Nasr, whose *Heart of Islam* remains a seminal text for Muslims and non-Muslims alike.[2] "For Islam," Nasr writes, "as for all authentic traditions, the goal of religion is to save the human soul and consequently establish peace and justice in society so that people can live virtuously and live and die 'in peace'" (221). Where within ISIS—or within Assad's Ba'athist regime, for that matter—do we see this "authentic . . . goal" pursued? As the Quran declares, "God guideth him who seeketh His pleasure unto paths of peace" (5:16).

God does not guide violence-driven radicals onto paths of war, though they conduct their acts of terror under the banner of jihad. Here, too, theirs is a gross distortion of the true Islamic teachings. The term "jihad" implies exertion and striving and struggle—but for what? The Muslim is called to defend his or her faith, but it is a "spiritual warfare" to which the jihadist is rightly called. As Nasr notes, "to overcome ignorance and to attain knowledge" is jihad "in its highest form" (260). And "the peace one seeks," Nasr continues, "comes through exertion on the path of God and striving to act according to His will" (260). I don't see ISIS terror or Ba'athist oppression as the sort of "striving" that leads the faithful, obedient Muslim to God's peace.

I'll have more to say about these themes, since they're unavoidable in a memoir about living and teaching in Assad's Syria. But let me quote one final passage, a hadith or saying of the Prophet (peace be upon him) that expresses the spirit of my own understanding:

> After the great battle of Badr, which was crucial to the survival of the newly born Islamic community . . . the Prophet, after having achieved victory, said, "You have returned from the lesser jihad to the greater (akbar) jihad." When asked what the greater jihad was, he said, "It is the jihad against your passionate souls." (Nasr 260)

It is in commitment to this personal, internal jihad that I have turned to writing. It is only by means of this "greater jihad" that the "lesser jihad" of blind violence can be cured. It is to this personal, internal jihad that I dedicate this book.

A second narrative interwoven through this memoir is a broader history of the Middle East after World War II, when the "warring twins" of Syria (est. 1946) and Israel (est. 1948) were given birth. This history is vital to understanding present-day Syria and its problems. I know that many readers will already possess a version of this history. It will be curious to compare my own experience and understanding of this history against the version most Americans have received via textbooks and popular media. Living in Assad's Syria, after all, is different from reading about it or watching it on American television.

You'll note that I've written, "Assad's Syria." Whereas Syria is the name of my native country, "Assad's Syria" is an ideological construct. Growing up under Hafez al-Assad, I was taught that the "eternal President" and the nation were one. The textbooks and newspapers of my youth never wrote of "Syria" merely. I lived and have taught, not in the Middle East simply, but within a repressive *ideology*.

The third and fourth narratives—family biography and personal memoir—are also interwoven. But there are differences between biography and memoir, as I've learned in writing. I can try to get "inside the heads and the hearts" of family members as they pass through their own trials, but what I "know" about their interior lives remains a mixture of empathy and imagination. In contrast, I can present a running record of my own thoughts, reflections, and reactions to current events—to the here-and-now of life, both here in Milwaukee, Wisconsin, and in Damascus, Syria.

Even as I write, I find myself living in two worlds simultaneously—and perhaps more than two, since the Damascus that I knew is not Damascus as it currently is and as it is coming-to-be. The whole of the Middle East is in the throes of change. It's hard to write in the past tense exclusively while a part of one's world changes drastically and daily.

As I've come to understand it, autobiography states the facts of one's life, whereas memoir states the truths. I write, not simply to say what has happened factually to me, my family, my faith, and my native land both in the past and just yesterday. I write, more importantly, to understand what has happened to me, my family, my faith, and my native land. And, most importantly, I write to be understood as an Islamic physician, medical ethicist, humanitarian—and Syrian refugee.

The story of my life has little human meaning or importance, unless another person bears witness to it. So, here I am. Look at me—a refugee from the Ba'athist regime, one voice from among the four million Syrians who have fled since 2011, scattering throughout the Middle East, Europe and, in my case, the United States. The United Nations High Commissioner for Refugees (UNHCR) confirms that figure, of which half are children. A 2014 European Union report on refugees counts another nine million Syrians displaced from their homes. My story is my own—and, as I've noted, I've felt the need to leave my native Syria twice, temporarily in 1988 and then for good in 2010. But there are millions of other stories of those millions of others who have lost their homes and livelihoods and have become voiceless, as good as forgotten. After all, Western media has kept its cameras trained on the politicians, the terrorists and the rebels. Rarely has it visited the refugee and displacement camps. Perhaps now, with the arrival of ISIS, this silence can be corrected.

Call me an émigré if you wish, a proud Syrian-American. It's only after I began writing this book that I've learned to call myself a refugee. After all, I had the means and the family connections to leave Syria in safety, and I left Syria of my own accord, bringing my wife and eventually my parents with me to America. (God bless America! When I was first drafting this very paragraph, the Fourth of July was just a few days away and I could hear the crackle of evening fireworks.) I do not bear the physical scars that many refugees do. I did not suffer the indignity of forced flight, with the crackle of gunfire behind me. Nor did I leave all worldly possessions behind—I left much behind, but not everything. No, what allows me to call myself a refugee is the recognition that I cannot go back. I am not welcome in Bashar al-Assad's Ba'athist Syria. I cannot go home. I love America and a part of me lives here in peace, but a part of me is homeless.

I wrote above that "I find myself living in two worlds simultaneously." I have to qualify that now. What I mean is that I live part of my life as a pediatric neurologist—first in Springfield, Missouri, and now in Milwaukee, Wisconsin—and part of my life as a Damascene refugee. If you asked me which of these worlds is "more real," I couldn't give you an easy answer. For each one of us, our worlds are material, physical, intellectual, psychological, emotional, spiritual, social, cultural. At any moment I can be intellectually in Milwaukee and emotionally in Damascus, socially in America and culturally in Syria. I have a head and I have a heart. I have a past and a present. I have memories and dreams, hopes and fears. All that should explain how I can live "in two worlds simultaneously" while being banished from the one where I was born and raised.

I stated that there were five narratives interwoven in this book. History, both recent and past, family biography, and memoir make four. And the fifth I've already alluded to. It's the self-conscious process of writing—of using writing to discover and reflect and reveal. I began by wanting to write and not knowing how or where to start. I started off, but didn't know where I was going. I found promising paths, but couldn't stay on them. I began wandering back and forth—reading and rereading, writing and rewriting. I did not know that writing was a conversation with the self—and an intense conversation, at that.

As I write, I find myself talking to myself, questioning my assertions and answering my questions. With each paragraph, I create readers and imagine their responses. I become my own reader and critic. I've had help in the writing and I needed it. Several friends lent me their minds, not to mention their skills as professional writers and editors. But, from start to finish, it is to WD Blackmon that I owe this little book. He took me under his wing—me, an amateur whose native language is Arabic, not English. We worked as one, emphatically, giving ourselves twelve months to produce a text that would normally take three-to-five years to produce. At least, that's what a press editor told me. (I think he was impressed by the speed of our work—and, I hope, by the timeliness and merit of the subject.)

Joined by a friend or two and family, we would sit around the table in my apartment or in the café at the local Barnes & Noble Bookstore and talk. I admit, I'm a good talker. They'd listen to a story or two and ask questions. Then they'd send me home with several writing assignments. I'd do the best I could, but my writing never seemed equal to my talking. I'd email WD my assignments and he'd rewrite and expand them, sending them back to me with more questions and requests for names, dates, and details—always more details.

When I got the first rewrite back, I felt guilty that a friend had made so much of the so little that I had given him. "Whoa, can you do this?" I asked him, naively: "Can I put my name on something that has so many of your words?"

"But, these are your thoughts," was his response. "This is what you told us. You'll learn as you go and, in time, you'll find your voice; until then, my job is to clothe your thoughts in Good Old American English and help you fill in the gaps."

"Okay," I said, "do as you will with me, my friend." I've just glanced back through our early email correspondence, to see what progress I've made. In one of the earliest emails, my friend wrote, "We have to talk more—a lot more—so that I can 'live inside you' and write the truth from your perspective." And so we did talk a lot more and, in the meantime, I wrote more and more. "You're getting better at this," he wrote a few weeks later—and I was feeling better about the process, since I had the final say in revision.

"You're a writer now," was his final pronouncement.

"And that's because of you, my friend," was my humble and heartfelt response.

I cannot thank WD enough for giving more than a year of his professional life to this memoir. Many of the idioms and turns of phrase came from his keyboard, but I'm content to say that the sentiments are mine and that I take responsibility for the whole.

* * *

I have a few further acknowledgments and disclaimers. I've written above that "my story is my own." And that's true, to an extent. I'm not the first Muslim to embrace the study of biomedical ethics and to publish in the field.[3] Still, "there are very few sources in Arabic or Persian devoted to biomedical issues, whether from the classical or the modern period"—so writes my fellow physician, Abdulaziz Sachedina, in his book-length discussion of Islamic biomedical ethics.[4] Dr Sachedina's thesis—to which I give my hearty agreement—is that "Muslim physicians must regard illness not merely as a physical phenomenon, but also as one with psychological and spiritual implications." He continues:

> [I]n Islam, medicine, hygiene, and communal health practices have religious implications as guidelines for good living according to God's will. . . . Medical doctors are exhorted to work sincerely under the guidelines of the Shari'a, to avoid all temptations to personal arrogance or greed, and to resist various social pressures that might conflict with their calling. Medical caring and curing should therefore be practiced in a climate of piety and awareness of the presence of God.[5]

If only Syrian health care proved faithful to this code! But my personal experience has been otherwise. The "pressures" of Ba'athism place politics before patient care—and the entire system, from med school professor down to the private practitioner, is riven by "arrogance" and "greed." Are there exceptions? Yes, of course. I know many Syrian physicians who practice the healing arts dutifully, intelligently, and piously. But in Assad's Syria, it's the exception that proves the rule.

I thank Scott C Davis of Cune Press for his savvy in publishing and for his unwavering commitment, not just to this present memoir, but to Middle Eastern affairs generally. Without independent presses like Cune, the full story of Syria would never be told. And I'd like to thank the many Americans—patients and colleagues, friends and casual acquaintances—whose conversations are recorded in the following chapters. Of course I can only approximate the conversations that I've had with different people over the years. In some cases, I've conflated these conversations, giving all the pertinent "arguments" to a composite figure—a "man on the street," so to speak. You cannot be Muslim in America without confronting the same questions on the same topics over and over again. With the help of my writer-friend, I've done my best to represent these topics within the conventions of memoir-writing. I've sought help in fact-checking everything presented as factual and in distinguishing fact from belief and opinion. But, again, for the sake of other people's security, I've walked over the terrain of Assad's Syria without leaving tracks. If I've left out some names or left in a few misspellings, I've had my reasons for doing

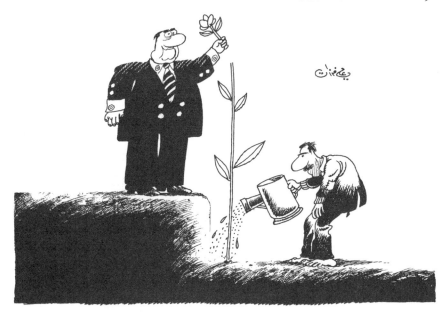

so—and, in so doing, I've stayed within the conventions of memoir-writing. So my writer-friend tells me, and I have no reason to disbelieve him.

May God grant peace, prosperity, and hope to all who read this book within the spirit in which it was written. I do not ask readers to agree with me on every point. My one request is that readers seek simply to understand me and to understand why I write and believe and profess what I do. From an ethical standpoint, understanding precedes agreement. If we all made mutual understanding a civic priority, there would be much less conflict in the world. To quote from the Quran (60:7):

> It may be that Allah will bring about love between you and those of them with whom you are now at enmity . . . . Allah forbids you not respecting those who have not fought against you on account of your religion, and who have not driven you out from your homes, that you be kind to them and deal equitably with them. Surely, Allah loves those who are equitable.

As an Islamic physician, medical ethicist, humanitarian, and Syrian refugee— and let me now add, as a fellow American—I take solace in these holy words.

1
A Letter from the Mossad

Anas narrates: "I heard the Prophet, peace be upon him, saying . . . 'When I afflict a servant of mine with respect to his two most beloved things (meaning his eyes), and he endures it patiently, I grant him paradise in return.'"

—Hadith, Fiqh us-Sunnah

My father was good at hiding the truth from us. It was November, 1972, and it had been close to three weeks since my brother, Samer, and I had last seen our mother.

"Your mother's gone to visit your grandmother Shaheera and aunt Hiyam in Jordan," my father had announced to us some twenty days ago.

"Why didn't she take us with her?" asked my brother back then, whining. My mother's family—our grandmother and uncles and aunts, with their children—lived in Amman. My brother and I were living with our mother in Beirut, where she had gotten a job. Our father was living and working in Damascus. We should have wondered why he had arrived in Beirut hurriedly and unannounced, leaving his work behind.

"She has business in Jordan. Don't worry," was my father's response, curt and explanatory though hardly comforting. I was seven at the time, my brother nine. We had travelled and moved several times over the past few years as my father and, later, my mother and father both looked for work. It was not unusual for her to travel. But why didn't she take us with her? And why had she been away so long?

My brother and I didn't worry, much. Personally, I hadn't yet learned how to read my father's anxieties. Usually, when he was happy his face showed it. And when he was angry his face showed it. And, usually, his words reflected his emotions. But, for the past twenty days, there was a grim fixity in my father's face. His words to us were kind and occasionally commanding, but they seemed overly matter-of-fact, as if flattened in intonation and affect. As an adult, I know that this was part of his coping. It helped him get through the business of the day, even as the world crumbled around him.

Neither my brother nor I had as yet caught on. Neither of us had a personal history of tragedy, so it wasn't yet in our natures to be anxious or afraid. I missed my mother tremendously. But I didn't fear for her. And then one evening in November, 1972, as Samer and I sat down at the dinner table, a crack opened in my father's façade.

"Kids," he said, "your Mom has had an accident while returning from Jordan and we're going to go see her tomorrow." Despite my father's faltering voice, Samer and I still didn't realize that the life of our family had shifted in a terrible way. We looked at each other and back at our father, whose eyes were fixed on his dinner plate. No further explanation was forthcoming.

"Dad, is Mom okay?" Samer asked, breaking the silence.

"Everything's going to be okay," was our father's non-answer: "Both of you go to bed after supper and be ready tomorrow when I call for you." That was how my personal lesson in shock and grief began.

It was past noon by the time the taxi picked us up. I had spent a restless night fighting off confusion and my growing fears, so I was scarcely attentive to the taxi ride, which took us through downtown Beirut. Street repairs and construction—rather, the tearing down of bombed-out buildings—made for traffic snags, though the street scenes didn't hold my interest as they normally would. In time, the taxi stopped and we got out. My eyes stayed pretty much on the back of my father's coat as we walked under a canopy, through glass doors, into a lobby, toward and away from a desk, down a hall, into an elevator, and out of the elevator—where I found myself standing in a corridor in the American University of Beirut Hospital.

As a child, the strangeness of certain places leaves visceral memories. I remember the hallway itself, painted a pastel mint-green. But, more than the sight, it's the smell that has haunted me since. Weird and alien to me, it was the first time in my life I had smelled anything like it, though it wouldn't be the last. Despite the strange setting, I was longing to see my mother after missing her so much for so long.

After walking some ways down the corridor, my Dad slowed down and announced, "Here's your mother's room." He meant the next room just ahead of us, but I turned immediately to the left, to look into the room we were just then passing. Contained within the room's pale green walls was a woman lying in bed, her face turned sideways toward the door, her eyes closed. A white blanket covered her, except for her legs. Some sort of box or wooden frame had been placed above her legs, over which a green sheet had been placed.

The strangeness of the sight stopped me in my tracks.

"Tarif!"

My father's voice urged me along but, at his voice, the woman awoke and our eyes met. My heart exploded in my chest and the explosion echoed in my ears. For the briefest of moments, we stared at each other. I do not know why her silent stare frightened me, but it did. It's as if her eyes, startled into wakefulness, were asking questions of me that I didn't know how to answer. Some days later, after I had gotten over some of the shock, I got up the courage to ask my father what I had seen. "Her legs are burned," he said, "and the box keeps the sheets from touching them, causing pain." Here, too, he knew more than he spoke.

"*Tarif!*"

Startled by my father's sharpened voice, I jumped back, almost tripping Samer who was walking behind me. Again, I did not know what I had just seen. Something had happened to the woman. Yes, accidents do happen. That was one of the platitudes that my father tried comforting us with on the way to hospital. But what sort of accident was this? It would be years before I could hazard an answer.

My mother's room was next. In it was a woman lying in bed, wrapped in sheets, with white cloth of some sort covering most of her face. These were the gauze bandages I would grow so familiar with over the next few years, but they were strange to me back then. My Dad shepherded us up close to the woman, pushing us past our natural reticence.

She seemed to grow agitated, though her movements were small, as if inhibited by the bandages. She did not speak, but she managed to raise her left arm toward Samer. I stood on her right side. That strange smell again, striking harder still.

With the three of us stationed around the bed, my father said, "Go on, get close to your Mom and give her a kiss."

As if in a dream, I looked from her to my father to my brother. Tears were welling up in Samer's eyes. "No!" Samer cried out, "*this* is not my mother!"

His crying grew desperate, causing a commotion on the hospital floor. Doctors and nurses rushed to the bedside and I was pushed out onto the balcony to make room for the medical staff.

So, on a brisk November afternoon I found myself standing alone on a hospital balcony overlooking the city of Beirut. And there, for the first time in my life, I called out to God. I remember the moment with terrific clarity. Although totally lost as to what was happening, I feared for my mother's life. "Please," I pleaded, "don't take my Mom." My prayer was answered.

* * *

How does a woman—a mere office secretary, someone trying to make a life for her two sons and husband—get caught up in the world's violence? Though years later, I can piece together parts of the puzzle. Here's how it happened for my mother.

The month prior—on September 4, 1972—the peaceful celebrations of the Munich Olympic Games had been shattered by political kidnapping and assassination. Eight members of Black September, a well-trained militant wing of the Palestinian Liberation Organization—the PLO—broke into the Olympic compound where Israeli athletes were staying, taking hostages and demanding the release of 234 Palestinians being held in Israeli jails. The Israeli Prime Minister, Golda Meir, refused to negotiate. Such refusal was official Israeli policy. Eleven athletes and five attackers died in the stand-off when German sharpshooters bungled a rescue attempt. The three surviving Black September commandos were jailed, but the September 29 hijacking of a Lufthansa jet led German authorities to release them in a trade.

Immediately and in secret, Golda Meir organized Operation Wrath of God, whose mission was to hunt down and kill the surviving attackers and anyone known or suspected of having aided in their attack. Spearheaded by the Mossad, Israel's equivalent of the American CIA, Operation Wrath of God began immediately and continued for two decades. Even to this day, I ask: "What did my mother do to earn the Wrath of God?"

Little did my family suspect that she would be among the first, though hardly the last, of the Operation's "collateral damage." That's a phrase that I've heard on American television when innocent civilians die in a military operation. So, let me describe the nature of my mother's "collateral damage."

My mother had moved from Damascus, Syria, to Beirut, Lebanon, where she took a job as secretary to Mr Nizar Azem, a successful businessman from an aristocratic Syrian family. Mr Azem was heavy set, with curly hair and a lazy eye. He was well-connected—and well-to-do. And he paid my mother well—far better than what my father was able to earn as a bank employee for the Ba'ath socialist government back home.

As a secretary, my mother's tasks were typical. Answering the phone and filing correspondence. Her boss did business with Rafiq al-Natsheh. The Hebron-born Natsheh worked previously in the Qatari Ministry of Education but had recently joined up with the PLO. And he would rise in the PLO ranks, joining the Fatah Central Committee in 1980. In 1998, he was appointed

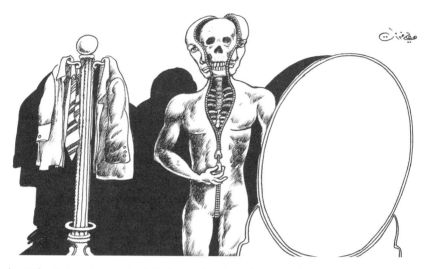

the Palestinian Authority Minister of Labor. In 2002, he became Minister of Agriculture. But all this lay in the future. Back in 1972, I remember him as a large man, mustached and balding, who came regularly to visit my mother's boss.

Mr Natsheh—or should I say, Dr Natsheh, given his political science PhD from the University of Moscow—began bringing his mail with him and asking my Mom to open it. He was a big man, as I've noted, and he threw his weight around. I've since learned that that's a habit of petty politicians in the Middle East. It's a given that power and wealth go hand-in-hand, and both are flaunted.

In sum, Rafiq al-Natsheh had become a target of the Israeli Mossad. He must have known that. In fact, the polite, lazy-eyed Mr Azem must have known that, as well. But my mother didn't know that. My mother was not a politician. Her concerns were more mundane, to put food on the table and clothe her children. And, despite recent world events, she didn't think much about the PLO operating in Lebanon at the time.

In all honesty, my mother hated the PLO whose leader, Yasser Arafat, had been vying with King Hussein for control of Jordan. And, in September, 1970—two years prior to the Munich games—the PLO raised the stakes with a series of plane hijackings and the planned assassination of the popular Hashemite king. PLO ambitions in Jordan ended in 1970, when Hussein's army broke the back of the PLO's military, expelling Arafat's forces. Retreating to Lebanon, what remained of the PLO's forces turned to terrorist operations exclusively, naming itself Black September after the 1970 hijackings.

My mother and grandmother were both Jordanian and both adored the

Hashemite King Hussein bin Talal. Among Arab leaders of his generation, he was moderate and in many ways enlightened. Yes, my mother and grandmother adored King Hussein. And they hated Yasser Arafat.

In preparing to write this memoir, I've asked my mother to tell me as much as she remembers about the day she opened Mr Natsheh's mail. She's a little more willing to speak about it now than in the past and she speaks about it almost matter-of-factly, as if the passing decades have made it seem more commonplace, just "a fact of life" (at least, of her life). As a physician I have, of course, heard people complain about their injuries and wounds, but rarely will they talk about them intimately, in the ways that they actually experienced them.

So, here's how I reconstruct the scene. Although it pains me, I can imagine the seconds before she opened the letter, sitting at her secretary's desk on a day otherwise much like any other. I wonder about the worries of her day, what may have crossed her mind, her daydreams even. There are so many ironies in that awful moment.

My mother arrives at the office, sitting down in her chair and sliding her legs under the desk. (While her sitting down protected her lower body, it also brought her chest and face closer to the blast.) She scans the mail sitting on her desk and picks up a pair of scissors. I've tried to reenact this moment myself, to get a "feel" for the scissors in my hand. In smaller right-handed scissors, you put your index finger through the bottom finger ring and your thumb through the top ring. But I'm assuming she used a larger pair of utility scissors, in which case the middle finger nestles inside the finger ring while the index finger sits outside on a curved finger rest. Right now, I'm holding such a pair of utility scissors. They rest loosely and fairly lightly in my right hand, opening and closing smoothly, ready to do their job.

Now I see my mother at her desk, holding the scissors in her right hand as she sorts through the pile of mail. A piece catches her attention. It's addressed to Rafiq al-Natsheh and the handwriting is sloppy, written in smudgy green ink. The green ink and the smudges strike her as unprofessional. She picks the letter up in her left hand and positions the scissors' blades on the envelope's right edge, so as to slice through the merest centimeter.

A phone call interrupts her. With the letter's edge suspended between the scissor's blades, she reaches with her left hand to the telephone, lifting the bulky receiver to her ear. It's a friend, calling to tell her that a man had been killed that day by a letter bomb. "Be careful!" was her friend's advice. As the phone call draws my mother's attention away from the envelope, she raises up and turns her face slightly to the left, as if to listen more intently. It turns out

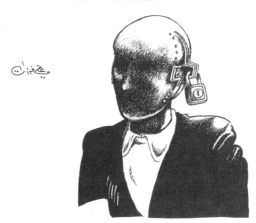

that this slight turn protects the left side of her face while exposing her right side fully to what happens next.

As she speaks, the letter sits to her right, one side resting on the desk top, the other suspended between the scissor's blades. Absentmindedly, her right hand begins to close, carrying the blades through the envelope. It takes a split second for the letter bomb to detonate and my mother's world to change.

Think, if you will, about the shock of a trauma that hits in an instant, without warning. Time slows, and our perceptions change in the midst of such injury. At first, one might not feel fear. One might not feel pain. It's in dire moments like these when we sense that we dwell in our bodies but that our consciousness—our blessed souls—transcend our mortal bodies. In effect, we become spectators—bystanders—witnessing our bodies' material ruin. As a physician, I have watched people gaze into their wounds with an almost childlike wonderment. Of course, the pain comes soon enough, bringing us back into our bodies and aware of our suffering.

Others in the office hear the explosion, but it is the sensation of light and pressure, not of sound, that dilates my mother's perception. It begins with a bright and intense flash, and the force is irresistible and all-encompassing. Her hand being closest to the blast, her right middle finger is blown off up to the first knuckle. I assume that the scissor's finger ring protected the knuckle itself. Her index finger is mangled but will be surgically repairable.

As the explosion mangles her hand, a blast of burning embers slams against her chest, neck, and the right side of her face. The fact that part of the letter bomb lay on the desk might seem to have lessened its blow. Had she held it in both hands, she would have taken its full force in her face. But now the bomb's force digs into the surface of the desk, sending up a second wave of wood-splinter shrapnel. This next image is gruesome: blood and shreds of clothing are splattered about. It's agonizing to imagine my mother's blood and flesh turned into human shrapnel.

It's the embers and splinters embedded in my mother's face that cause the greatest ruin. Her right eye is punctured and closes. It will never open again.

The rest is chaos. In a panic, coworkers rush into the office, neglecting their own safety. There's confused shouting and groans of empathy. There's a frantic phone call for an ambulance, followed by a phone call to my father. My mother is now lying on the floor in shock, though she recalls a curious detail. As if oblivious to the situation and her condition, she gives orders to coworkers regarding the rest of the day's work—always dutiful, always the secretary.

The wait for the ambulance seems an eternity. At last, it arrives. On their way to the hospital, paramedics inject morphine into her and prepare for the emergency room operation that is to come. The years to follow will be filled with forty more surgeries and never-ending therapy and anger and remorse, but for now the only fact that matters is that she is alive. My mother had survived the Mossad. Not many have.

* * *

As a seven-year-old, I understood next to nothing of all this. As an adult, I still don't understand much about that day. But here are some reflections.

First, it's hard to fathom that my mother could be treated as mere "collateral damage" in a war of terror between Palestinians and Israelis. In one respect, the Mossad failed in its mission: Rafiq al-Natsheh was still alive and safe. In another, it had succeeded, since its aim was terror, as well as revenge. The bombing indeed brought terror into that Beirut office, and, in a sense, to Israel's enemies in general and to anyone who lived or worked with or near them.

And what of the woman with charred legs in the hospital room next to my mother's? She, too, was most probably a piece of "collateral damage," though the bomb that ruined her legs likely arrived via an Israeli jet rather than the post. I know now that the Israeli Air Force bombed refugee camps in Lebanon and Syria on September 8, 1972—four days after the Munich kidnapping. Ten suspected PLO positions were targeted and the casualties, both military and civilian, numbered in the hundreds. Many of these were treated in hospitals in Beirut.

Acts of blood vengeance are as old as humanity—witness Cain and

Abel—and defy the ways of peace as set forth in the Quran. Our highest calling, whether Jew or Christian or Muslim, is to bring peace into the world. The true jihad, as recounted in the Quran, is an internal struggle. It is the inferior, ungodly aspects of ourselves that we are called to conquer. To be filled with hatred and blood lust, to feed off of lack of forgiveness, makes us enemies of God. Hatred and blood lust poison the soul. Worse, they are addictive. The desire for vengeance can take over the mind and spirit of an individual, a community, a nation.

As powerful as it was, the Mossad's letter bomb wasn't strong enough to kill with any surety. Perhaps its purpose was to maim and blind, to set a living example for all to see: *This is what happens when you attack Israel.* And that's why I would describe this as an act of terror rather than of eye-for-an-eye blood revenge. In blood revenge you aim to kill the body. In terrorism you aim to kill the will and the soul.

It was a *message* that the Mossad was sending, and even if the wrong person opened the letter, the message was received: "There is no safe haven. There is no peace." And here's what I find most grievous. Rafiq al-Natsheh knew the ways of the Mossad and knew what to expect. It was a cowardly deed, to have an innocent Jordanian woman open his mail, knowing full well that a bomb could arrive in his name. He had to have known it. He *knew* it. And I suppose that my mother's boss, the charming Mr Azem, knew it, too. My mother did not. She had no reason to suspect this. She was just working in Lebanon, trying to feed her family. I have repeated this litany to myself for decades.

Did I forgive Mr Natsheh? For decades, I couldn't. Did I forgive the man who sent the bomb that maimed my mother's face, blinding her in her right eye? Over the years, I've wished for the bomb's makers and the logistics planners responsible to be blinded, tortured, and killed a thousand times over in a thousand horrific ways.

Can I forgive the bomber? I can, and I must. I do. But it wasn't always this way for me.

Some time in the late 1970s—while I was a student at Al-Thaqafi Secondary School in Damascus—I remember watching an American movie in a local theatre. It was about Black September. A web-search tells me that it must have been *21 Hours at Munich*, a 1976 made-for-TV movie that was released in several foreign countries—including Syria, it seems. I've seen a poster for it on the Internet: "The most violent episode in the history of terrorism," the poster proclaims. Without denying the wasteful violence of this "episode," a declaration of that sort sounds so childishly naïve. What about

Kristallnacht of November 8-9, 1938, when 30,000 German and Austrian Jews were rounded up and thrown in concentration camps—a mere taste of the mind-numbing mass-produced and mechanized violence to come? Over that evening in 1938, one hundred European Jews were killed in their own native land by their fellow Germans and Austrians. Their homes, businesses, schools, and synagogues were ransacked, torched, destroyed. I could name other acts of terror against Jews, acts of violence reaching back hundreds and even thousands of years. But, in 1976, when that American movie poster was printed, "The most violent episode in the history of terrorism" had been reduced to an Arab-Israeli affair.

When the PLO commandos killed the Israeli athletes, the movie audience in Damascus cheered—and, sad to say, I cheered along. At that moment, I was not thinking of my mother's scarred face, of her suffering in retaliation. My cheering was visceral—a knee-jerk reaction. After all, I had been born and raised in a country whose people had been taught to hate Israelis, all of them. Hatred of Israel was part of the Ba'athist school curriculum. We were taught how horrible the Israelis were, how they stole our land and killed our women and children. During the 1972 Munich Games, Syrians cheered when they watched the news on TV. And here we were, a few years later, watching that movie, cheering again.

I have grown over the decades, having become a practitioner of medicine and a student as well as a teacher of ethics. And I have delved more deeply into the true Islamic teachings. So I've come to regret my feelings and actions in that movie theater on that afternoon in Damascus. The killing of Israeli athletes was a terrible act against humanity, against Islam, against God.

Recently, I bought a copy of *Life* magazine from 1972 that details the Black September attack. It's one thing to read about history in a textbook. It's another thing to read it "raw," as it unfolded in popular media. The cover shows the victims marching in the Munich opening ceremony. As I look one by one at their faces, I can imagine the sorrows of the mothers and the fathers, the spouses and the children they left behind. Their sorrows are no different from the sorrows of Palestinian men, women, and children who, over the years, have lost loved ones to political violence. You can learn a lot from an old *Life* magazine.

2
A Care-Free Childhood
(Blasted by Carnage & Bracketed by War)

You shall certainly be tried and tested in your possessions and in your lives. And you will certainly hear much that will grieve you . . .

—Quran 3:186

"I would have killed myself if it wasn't for you, my children," my mother told me when I was sixteen.

"Oh, Mom, please—don't talk like that." What else is a teenager to say when words are dropped like a bombshell, without warning? I don't remember what we had been talking about, what might have led her to say such a thing. I don't think she said it out of anger or self-pity, both of which can motivate a stereotypical "mother's complaining." Besides, I had come to think of her as a strong woman, an independent, accomplished, successful woman.

"You are old enough to hear this," she said in reply, "and so I tell you this now." Actually, I wasn't old enough. I was old enough, perhaps, to hear the words—which she would repeat many times over the next four decades—but it would take years before I understood the full meaning behind the words. What she was saying was that there are some things more important than one's own life and, for her, being a mother was one of those things. She was no longer living for herself. Though she had survived, the letter bomb had effectively killed that person that she had imagined she was or had aspired to be. Perhaps, along with her outward beauty, it had stolen her hope. Whatever the Mossad's letter had taken from her or killed in her, she was now living *for us*.

Reflecting back, I realize that my mother was kept alive by coming straight home from the hospital and cooking and caring for us as best she could. I remember her trying to sweep the kitchen, holding the broom in her left hand—her right having been mangled—with thick gauze bandages wrapped across the right side of her face, covering the socket of her lost right eye. I remember her wearing a shiny green satin robe when she first came home, her face raked and pock-marked with grayish abrasions.

I was stricken back then when I looked at her. She had been so beautiful. Now, I realize that what she was doing for Samer and me was as beautiful as anything I have experienced on this earth. Even now, some forty-two years later, I am reminded of this every time I hug her. And I thank God that I can be so close to her, now that she's living in the same apartment complex in the same city as I am. I can return to her some of the loving care that she has lavished on her husband and children.

After the destruction, of course my mother couldn't keep her job. So we moved back to Damascus, where my father had been working for the government-owned Commercial Bank of Syria. Later my father became an employee of the Ba'athist Ministry of Economics and Trade. This might sound like a sweet political appointment, but my Dad "worked for peanuts," as they say in the States.

Following the lead of Egypt's secularist president, Gamal Abdel Nasser (1956-1970), the infrastructure of much of the Syrian economy had been nationalized. Nasser's Soviet-inspired policies and promotion of pan-Arab unity—culminating in the ill-fated United Arab Republic of Egypt and Syria (1958-1962)—promised much but delivered little for the average Syrian. My father told me that before Ba'athism restructured the nation's political economy, the Syrian pound was a healthy currency, at one time near in value to the US dollar. But inflation soon set in, and it has never abated. With civil war raging today, inflation has really skyrocketed. Now, it takes 375 Syrian pounds to buy one US dollar.

In 1961—the year before my parents married—my father had a promising career with the Arab Bank, the Middle East's largest private bank at the time. But the politics of nationalization would soon cost him his private-sector job and, by 1972, our little family was virtually bankrupted. That's why my mother took the job as secretary in Lebanon, to help our family make ends meet. But we soon found ourselves back in Syria, worse off for having lost her income, relying on help from relatives and living off Dad's pittance of a socialist government salary.

And it's not like my mother had simply to suffer through the initial blast and then learn to live with her disability. She had to suffer through some forty surgeries to repair at least some of the damage. I can't forget the procedures she underwent and how, as she lay on our living room couch, I stared wide-eyed while doctors changed the bloody, iodine-stained bandages on her face. I winced each time they cut and pulled one of many stitches. Though a physician by training, I still have that same nauseous, clenched feeling in my stomach when I think back on those moments.

* * *

Despite the horror that I've described, most of my early childhood comes back to me in a pleasant haze of contentment heightened by an occasional spice of ecstasy. I remember any number of horrific things happening, but they didn't seem to be happening to me, personally. I seemed to be an observer in each case, the one who was spared.

I don't recall much before the age of five, when we were living in Damascus in the late 1960s. I do remember a young servant, probably ten or eleven years old, whose name was Zainab. It was a custom back then to have a child from a poor country village move in with an urban family for a small salary, which was then given to the child's parents. So Zainab lived with us in our basement apartment on Cordoba Street in the Malki district. Back then, I didn't know the name of the street or the neighborhood. But I remember Zainab, because she used to play with my brother and me.

Other of my toddler "memories" are reconstructions from photographs. In the family photo album, there's a photo of me standing in the small backyard garden holding a big neighborhood cat. In another, I'm chasing after a neighborhood dog. There's another of me smiling in the lap of my paternal grandmother Farizeh. These photos show me as a chubby little guy. And no wonder, with all the food served at family gatherings.

Ah, the "haze of contentment" and "spice of ecstasy." In a toddler's world, *these* come from food and family! Of all my relations, it's my maternal grandmother, Jordanian born grandma Shaheera, who comes quickest (and most fondly) to mind. Short and stocky with dancing blue eyes, grandma Shaheera lived to cook for her husband, Subhi, her children (including my mother, Nawal), and her grandchildren. It was a beautiful part of growing up, the way we were welcomed into the homes of relatives where we were met by the smells of Middle Eastern cooking. I remember visiting grandma Shaheera in Amman after she was widowed and was living with my uncle Shafik's family. She would insist on us eating . . . and eating . . . and eating. Eating more meant you loved her more, and I loved her tremendously. The very names of the spices she used in her dishes sound like the refrain to a poem of my childhood:

Cumin, nutmeg, cardamom;
turmeric, caraway, aniseed;
allspice, cinnamon and saffron!

Oh, and add the tart juice of lemons.

As a child, I imagined that I could smell her home—that is, her home cooking—from miles away. (I swear I can smell those same spices now, decades later, from almost seven thousand miles away.) And then the next day, after gorging at grandma's, we'd visit my mother's sister, aunt Hiyam. And all of us—Samer and I, along with my aunt's five children—would gather around her big kitchen table. How blessed we were! We'd eat and laugh, throwing jokes around the table well into the night. When I think about my childhood, these are the moments I want to remember.

As a toddler, I couldn't have known that the world was changing around us. That my father's career in private banking would put him on the "losing side" of pan-Arab nationalism. That his employer at the Bank was none other than Nazim al-Qudsi, onetime President of Syria. That al-Qudsi would be deposed and driven into exile. And that, with my father's career in shambles, the search for work would lead our family from Syria to Morocco, back to Syria, back to Lebanon, then back to Syria.

In 1970, when I was five years old, my father was hired as an accountant. It was at a factory that made socks, and the factory was in Tangier, Morocco. With his game face on, he announced the move as an adventure—as if Tangier were the fairyland of North Africa. But going from the Bank to a Moroccan shoe factory must have insulted his pride, not to mention his wallet.

If I had been older, I might have appreciated the history and the culture: Morocco might well have proved the fairyland that my father described to us kids. But a five-year-old tends to focus on things close at hand. The house we rented was smaller than the apartment and we had no servant, though I do remember a woman named Raheemah who came every few days to bake bread for us.

Morocco was alien to me, and I felt lost—at times literally. It didn't help that I was just starting school, too. From my five-year-old point of view, it seemed that Moroccans treated children roughly. My father would raise his voice but rarely his hand against us, and he never sought to hurt us. My schoolteacher, on the other hand, was cruel. If someone misbehaved in class, he would tell four students to hold the miscreant on a table while he'd beat the kid's bare feet with a sturdy stick. He never hit me, though that may have been because I was Syrian—a "foreign guest."

But we weren't long in Morocco. After little more than a year my Dad lost his job, so we moved back to Damascus to stay with uncle Hisham. My father, mother, brother, and I lived together in one room. Being homeless in the Middle East isn't all that uncommon, though it increases one's sense of helplessness. As parents of two school-age children, my parents must have felt great anxiety—not to mention humility, in having to live off another's kindness. It was this pervasive anxiety that led my mother to take a job in Beirut as secretary to Mr Azem. Once she got this well-paying job, we felt our fortunes as a family improve, although I realize now that my father carried a burden of guilt, being unable to provide for his family as he had hoped. Again, that was in 1972, and I was seven at the time.

While my father was still hiding the truth from us, I'm sad to say that—being unaware of our Mom's condition—Samer and I had a terrific time of it. In place of our routine lives, we found ourselves invited to so many homes, with everyone so kind and caring, pampering us at every turn.

Mr Azem often invited us to supper. He was a wealthy man and his home was luxurious. Whenever I ate at Mr Azem's, I felt like a prince. It was during Ramadan, and there was so much sumptuous food spread out on that long, fancy table of his, including the sticky-sweet honey baklava I loved so much.

I don't remember much between our first visit to the hospital and the day when my mother was let out. I suppose I was in shock. I do remember my Jordanian grandmother and aunt visiting us in Lebanon, before we moved back to Damascus. One day aunt Hiyam took us to a movie theater. *Dr Zhivago* was the feature film, with subtitles in Arabic. Spectacular visually, filled with the strains of *Somewhere, My Love*—a song beautiful and sad—it showed trains screaming across a snowy Russian landscape. Tumultuous crowds were shot down by soldiers in the chaotic streets. Cossacks and uniformed cavalry thundered against foot soldiers and against each other, the clash of swords and volleys of gunshots and cannons echoing above the drifting smoke of battle. There was the good doctor passionately kissing the beautiful, fur-hatted young woman and then rushing off from her embrace to some new, desperate errand. And the toughest, cruelest officer of all wore an eye-patch, having been blinded in one eye. Not a great choice of movies for a traumatized child like me.

My mother told me later that, when they first took her into the Emergency Room at the University of Beirut Hospital, they refused to help her unless someone guaranteed the payments—which her boss did. Mr Azem had multiple business dealings across the Middle East. Among his trading partners were revolutionaries in the Yemeni Socialist Party—which had recently taken control of South Yemen—and their Lebanese allies in the PLO. Again, I'm not sure how much my mother could have known about Mr Azem's business partners. I do recall a man coming into my Mom's office one day. Two chairs had been placed on the far side of her desk. I was sitting in one, and the man came in and sat in the other next to mine. When I stood up, the man started stroking my hair with his one hand. His other hand was missing. My Mom told me later that Hafez al-Assad's one-time ally, the Egyptian President Gamal Abdel Nasser, had ordered the man's other hand plunged in boiling-hot oil. It never crossed my mind to ask, "Why?"

Of course, neither the Yemenis nor the PLO lifted a finger to help with my mother's medical bills. It's curious how life goes on when troubles strike other people elsewhere. I imagine that Mr Azem and Mr Natsheh both went home that night after the bombing and enjoyed their evening meals as best they could, taking in the sights and smells and conversation at the family dinner table. (I guess the same was true for Samer and me, except that we didn't know about the blast and we weren't the ones who had set our mother up for tragedy.)

Moving back to Damascus from Beirut, we found ourselves living in an apartment building owned by my maternal uncle, Shafeek. It was in the Malki neighborhood in the western part of the city, close to Mount Qasioun. Overlooking the ancient city, Mount Qasioun happened to be near where the New Shaab Presidential Palace would be built.

When we moved into the neighborhood, many of the roads were not yet paved. So at times I stood ankle-deep in mud waiting for the school bus to pick me up. (After a few years, I would graduate to the Al-Thaqafi School, which I could walk to—or ride to on my own, after I got my bike). The rooms in our apartment were cold, but we had a stove in the living room and I loved sitting close to it in winter, watching the flames behind the small smoky glass window. Sometimes my father would throw a piece of orange peel into the fire, so the room would be spiced by the scent of orange oil. Our apartment was on the third floor and consisted of five rooms plus one bathroom. My parents had to leave many times for Spain or Czechoslovakia to get the surgeries my Mom needed. At those times, one of our uncles would stay with us.

The bedroom that I shared with my brother was small, barely holding two beds and a cabinet for our clothes. Attached to our bedroom was a small balcony, on which were placed two children's study desks. I used to spend hours each day sitting at my balcony-desk, getting up only to eat or take a few minutes of rest. I studied hard and made it to the top of my class. And I loved being at the top of my class.

ريفقت

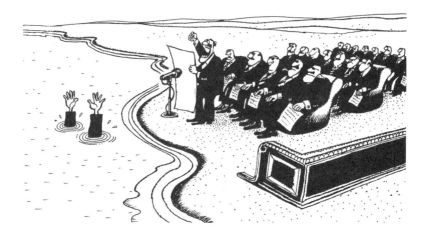

Throughout our public schooling, we wore military uniforms. This was one of many Soviet influences—as if we were Arab versions of Russian Young Pioneers. Each school morning we had to stand and salute the flag while reciting the Ba'ath Party pledge. There were thirty to forty kids in a typical elementary school class, with two students per desk. (Over the years, it inflated to three students per desk—and, now, with civil war raging, many schools across Syria have been razed to the ground.)

I always sat in the front row, concentrating fiercely on the teacher. I liked most of my teachers, and they liked me. I didn't make many friendships with the kids in my class, though I became close with two or three. With my short hair and big-framed glasses, I guess I'd be called a "nerd" nowadays.

I walked the streets of my neighborhood in the Malki district thousands of times. It seemed a blessing that President Hafez al-Assad was now living close by, since the whole area had grown. The streets were being paved and wealthy people were moving in, building and buying big homes.

With the passage of years, my mother's physical wounds healed and it came time for her heal emotionally, to get out of the house and regain some semblance of her former social life. So I began taking her to language classes at the French Cultural Center in Damascus. I was twelve at the time. Leaving our apartment, we'd walk the narrow cobblestone path down the hill to the Cultural Center. I'd take hold of her hand and lead her up old, broken stairs in the dim light. Around eight o'clock in the evening, after her two hours of lessons, I would fetch her back home. She began to make new female friends and I was happy to see her smile once more.

My mother was now ready for the next step in her recovery. Since our finances remained precarious, she would go back to work—but she resolved to work for no man. Set on being her own boss, she began trading Turkish goods in Syria, traveling to purchase the items herself. It was the late 1970s and Muslim women were not supposed to go out alone, traveling long distances by themselves. For a married woman, sitting next to male truck drivers for the 650-mile trip from Damascus to Ankara and back was unthinkable.

Outraged, many of our family's friends and acquaintances scolded my father, trying to shame him for giving my mother such freedom—especially since she was working with men who weren't our blood-relations. But my Dad didn't hold her back. He knew she needed her freedom. And she did well. The money we now had was thanks to her ingenuity and hard work. She even contracted with government agencies. I remember one particular bid that she won to supply doors from Turkey. Her courage, strength, and determination were inspiring.

Once a trip was completed, my mother would cook a feast for her Turkish business partners, both men and women. I loved talking to them and learning from them. For these visitors, the table would be set with a half-dozen or more dishes that made one's mouth water: *kibbeh* (fried croquettes stuffed with minced lamb), *fateh* (a spicy meat casserole with chickpeas and yogurt sauce, covered with toasted pine nuts), *makloubeh* (a casserole of meat, vegetables, and rice), *mansaaf* (sautéed lamb chunks in yogurt sauce, served over rice), *mehshi* (meat-stuffed eggplant), *fattoush* (toasted pita with mixed greens and vegetables), varieties of *kebab*—and all the yogurt, the cucumbers and tomatoes, the white cheese, rice, the ubiquitous olive oil.

As a young teenager, my own daily routine was simple. I'd go from home to school down a hill, passing through an area that had barricades on both sides of a street packed with the homes of high-ranking Syrians. There were security guards all around and brand-new cars everywhere, mostly black Mercedes with dark-tinted windows. You did not want to look around or up at the buildings and the guards, because of the fear that had been instilled in you over the years. At times you would glimpse the six- or seven-year-old son or daughter of one of these government officials. The security guards would run to open the car door, bowing and kowtowing to the brat as if their own lives depended on it. The rest of us neighborhood teens had so much hate for these kids, though our hatred mixed with fear of their guards.

Typically, these security guards were not well dressed. Most wore sandals made of rubber and, as a show of machismo, they left their shirts unbuttoned,

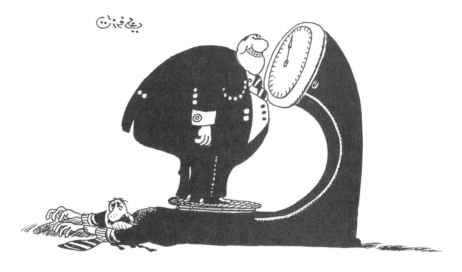

showing us far more than we wanted to see of their hairy chests and bulging bellies. Of course, their most prominent fashion accessory was the AK-47 slung over their shoulders. These guards were largely poor and uneducated and would likely have been sent off to the latest war front (or to our long-standing occupation of Lebanon), had they not landed this "plum" of a job.

It was my daily walk past the barricades and the security guards and the palatial homes that first caused me to question my faith in the Syrian government. Throughout our school years, we were taught the cult status of our President, the glory of the Ba'ath Party, and the praises of socialism. Though adult members of my extended family might grumble around the kitchen table, nothing in our public lives contradicted the cult status of our President, the glory of the Ba'ath party, and the praises of socialism. Not our teachers in "national education," not our textbooks, not our television, not our newspapers. But what I saw on my daily walk contradicted everything I was being taught by our teachers, textbooks, television, and newspapers.

It was at this time that I asked to join the Ba'ath Party, much to my father's dismay. I was thirteen and the principles of socialism—particularly the equitable distribution of resources (which justified the seizing of private property)—appealed to my youthful idealism. But if Ba'athist Syria (as we were told) was a socialist paradise, what my eyes showed me was far otherwise. In my very neighborhood, government cronies flaunted their wealth while the rest of us struggled to make ends meet. There was an elitism at play here, but one that I was not yet equipped to understand. All I knew, intuitively, was that something wasn't fair, something wasn't right.

Though my parents had instilled a strong work ethic in me and I felt driven personally to excel in my studies, I couldn't see any connection between hard work or industry and reward within the Ba'athist system. There was indeed a "reward system" in place, but when I glanced (furtively) at the men and their families who lived in the houses down the hill from our apartment and who drove in the black Mercedes and were protected by these brutish armed guards, all I saw was in their faces was hauteur, crassness, and indifference.

And then I confronted a cold fact, whose implication had been hiding from me. There were good reasons why I was taught to avoid eye contact with the armed guards and high-ranking government officials. The barriers in that neighborhood had been erected for a purpose. The Ba'ath Party was not, as I was taught, the great protector of the Syrian people. Years before the current civil war broke out, the Ba'athists were already barricading themselves from the people they were exploiting. With guns at the ready, they were suspicious—fearful, rather—of their own fellow citizens. For years, I had to walk past these barricades twice daily and be reminded of how, through the error of a casual sideways glance, I could be harassed or jailed—or, for all I knew, shot.

Though an important step, this was but the first step in my personal re-education. Though I was beginning to lose faith in Ba'athism and socialism, I did not yet understand the extent of the hypocrisies, the downright lies, the oppression, and the violence that the Assad regime visited daily upon the Syrian people. It was around age sixteen—about the same time that my mother confessed her early contemplations of suicide—that I began to see past the Ba'athist propaganda to a darker, unspoken truth. I began to question the official histories and the contemporary news reports, though I didn't know what to supply in place of those official histories and reports, since the world "out there," with its competing/alternative viewpoints, was forbidden territory and closed off from us.

* * *

So much for my early memories of home and school. Let me now give my early memories of war.

I remember nothing directly about the Six-Day War, since I was two years old at the time. Of course, being Syrian-born, I have not escaped its legacy. The Six-Day War has weighed heavily in the consciousness of Arabs in the Middle East since 1967, but especially before the Yom Kippur War of 1973. To steal a metaphor from English poet, Samuel Taylor Coleridge, the Six-Day War has hung like an albatross around Arab necks for all this time. It got a bit lighter after the Yom Kippur War, but it's still there, hanging like a dead weight.

I have come to blame Gamal Abdel Nasser, the Soviet-backed president-dictator of Egypt, for this military-political fiasco. Nasser was a powerful orator but a mediocre military strategist, and it was he who led the Arab coalition bent on the destruction of Israel. As if his own bungling wasn't bad enough, I've lived with rumors that the Egyptian Vice President and Deputy Supreme Commander, Abdel Hakim Amer, had become a hopeless drug addict. Amer's order to retreat from the Sinai sealed the Egyptian army's defeat and he (not Nasser) was popularly blamed for the disaster. Sacked within a month, Amer plotted a coup against his one-time ally. Arrested and accused, he took his own life by suicide.

As I've noted, Nasser wielded tremendous charisma. He could talk for hours, holding audiences spellbound. I've heard parts of his speeches and can attest to his skill. During his ascent to power—only a year or so before he became absolute ruler in name as well as in fact—he was giving a speech in Alexandria when an assassin from the Muslim Brotherhood, standing twenty-five feet away, fired eight quick shots at him. One can hear the crackle of gunshots in the recording, followed by screams and confused shouting. Miraculously, all eight shots missed. But, in the pandemonium, the crowd hadn't realized that Nasser wasn't struck by the gunfire. He didn't miss a beat. Raising his own voice above the din, Nasser built the assassination attempt into his speech, shouting out his willingness to shed blood for Egypt, even to die for Egypt, so that its people might gain their rightful place in the sun.

Before the Six-Day War, Nasser gave many speeches about destroying Israel and regaining Palestine. For pan-Arab audiences, these were no doubt compelling. Nasser demanded that the UN guards between Israel and its Arab neighbors be removed. When that was done, he began military maneuvers, and that's when Israel launched intense and simultaneous surprise attacks against Egypt, Jordan, and Syria. To the world at large it appeared that Nasser's military actions along the Egyptian-Israeli border led Israel to make pre-emptive strikes.

Now, however, we know that the Israeli attacks had been meticulously planned and coordinated in advance. Israel wanted buffers on every side against its most powerful Arab neighbors. The Sinai Peninsula from Egypt, the West Bank from Jordan, and the Golan Heights from Syria.

Looking back, it seems to me that Nasser's strongman posturing gave the Israelis the fig leaf they needed to portray their military action as defensive. Nasser gave speeches, but Israel took action. The Israeli air force destroyed most of Egypt's aircraft while they were still on the ground. Nasser said that he expected the Israelis to attack from one direction but they attacked from another. (Well, that explains it all, doesn't it?)

My father has since told me that, during the early hours and days of the war, the news media in Syria and Egypt consistently lied to the people, declaring that the combined Arab forces were winning and that most of Israel's air force and tanks had been destroyed. And when the truth was at last told, people throughout the Arab world were left in shock. The battles had all been lost. The vaunted Egyptian army was in retreat in the Sinai and tens of thousands of young men had been killed, wounded, or captured.

In a mere six days, between June 5 and June 10, the Israeli forces rolled over the armies of three great Arab nations at once—and made it seem like a breeze. Though outnumbered and spread out across three fronts, the Israeli forces managed to wrest the West Bank from Jordan, including the holy city of Jerusalem. From Egypt, the Israelis took the Gaza Strip and entire Sinai Peninsula. From Syria, the Israelis took the Golan Heights. Many thousands of people in these now-occupied lands left their homes and fled to neighboring states, especially Jordan, Syria, and Lebanon. Their flight added to the hundreds of thousands of refugees from Palestine, who had been homeless for two decades already.

I have to admit that my life under the Assads left me bitter. Even so, I still habitually viewed history through the distorted lens provided by Ba'ath doctrine. Despite Israel's devastating surprise attack, I have to admit that I always felt that, as Syrian Defense Minister during the Six-Day War, Hafez al-Assad should have paid the price for the loss of the Golan Heights—his political fortunes should have been ruined. Not only did Assad survive the debacle, he led a coup three years later to take sole power as president. Syria is officially a republic with an elected president. Under Assad, however, the Syrian government became more like an absolutist monarchy—a point that became clear after Hafez Assad's death, when the constitution was amended to allow his previously too-young son Bashar to become president.

The Egyptian President Nasser, too, survived. On June 9—the day before peace treaties were signed—Nasser came on TV and radio to take responsibility for the loss, declaring that he had resigned the presidency. Later in life, I listened to a recording. What struck me was the calmness of his delivery. It was a shrewd tactic, it turns out. Pouring onto the streets by the tens of thousands, the Egyptian people gave their resounding mandate that he stay in power. And he did so—though not for long, as he died within three years.

Given the Egyptian people's embrace of Nasser after this shocking defeat,

I'm left to wonder: Why, in the Arab world, do we glorify our leaders even when they bring such destruction upon their people? What would happen if an Israeli leader had suffered such loss? Would that nation clamor for his continued leadership? Of course not. The year after Israel was surprised by the Arab attack in the Yom Kippur War, for example, Golda Meir resigned in response to "the will of the people." Then again, there are multiple parties in Israel. In Syria, as in Saddam's pre-Gulf War Iraq, there's only the Ba'ath Party.

Syria's one-party system was built on an old Soviet model. And, to the extent that the Soviet model aims at maintaining and concentrating power, it has served the Assad family—first Hafez and, now, Bashar—in its will to survive. But personal loyalty is a strongly-held value in Arab culture, and loyalty to a politician or party invokes some of the psychology of family loyalty.

Over the centuries, Islamic culture has made vital contributions to science, logic, and philosophy. During the European Dark Ages, it was Islam that kept learning alive. And yet, the old tribal loyalties of many Arabs today make politics an affair of the heart and not of the brain. Beyond vested self-interest, that's the only explanation I can offer for those Syrians today who clamor, with such high zest, for the survival of Assad's murderous regime.

Let me add that Nasser's errors did not end with the Six-Day War. His nationalizing of land and major industries in Egypt and Syria destroyed much of the economic power of the private sector in these countries, Syria especially. Many smaller businesses went under, and those individuals to whom he gave power (either as bribery or a reward for loyalty) were skilled in corruption.

All this I came to learn in adulthood, after the fact. Nasser died of a heart attack in 1970, when I was five years old. It was with his successor, Anwar El Sadat, that my direct knowledge of war begins. Upon assuming the Egyptian presidency, Sadat continued Nasser's militaristic policies.

I was eight years old during the Yom Kippur War. In "round two" of the festering Arab-Israeli conflict, it was Egypt and Syria's turn to make a surprise attack. I remember dancing for joy with my brother in our Damascus home when we heard about the liberation of the Golan Heights. You'll remember that the Mossad had attacked my mother just twelve months prior. Her wounds were barely healed, so we rejoiced as Syrian forces sought revenge on our family's behalf.

Syrian newspapers printed photographs of Israeli jets shot down by Soviet-supplied SAM-2 and SAM-3 surface-to-air missiles. There was one photo that I remember vividly. It was of a charred Israeli pilot burned inside his crashed jet with chains wrapping him in his seat so that he could not escape.

I know what I saw as a child, so I've searched for corroboration. In his book, *No Victor, No Vanquished,*[6] British military journalist Edgar O'Ballance reports seeing a copy of a photo similar to the one I've described. He writes, "the Syrians allege that toward the end of the war, Israeli morale was so low that Israeli pilots had to be chained in their cockpits" (150). "But this," he continues, "can hardly be believed" (150), the implication being that such photos were staged or somehow doctored for propaganda. As an adult, I would prefer that such photos were doctored. The thought of anyone being chained to any instrument of war is repulsive to the core. But, again, this is what I was shown as a child, and it's not an image I can simply erase from my mind and memory.

While "round one" lasted six days, this second round lasted nearly three weeks, from October 6 to October 25, 1973. We felt its effects in Damascus. Though we had no shortage of food, our home lost running water and electricity many times throughout. Yet the outages seemed a small price to pay for the victory that, according to Syrian news, was immanent and inevitable. Through the first two weeks, all we heard of was victory—the recapture of the Golan Heights and of most of the Sinai Peninsula. But the tide of battle began to turn long before the news coverage changed.

As in the Six-Day War, the Yom Kippur War pitted American against Soviet military hardware and logistics. And, as the bullets and missiles began running out on either side, the two Cold War rivals raced to resupply their respective allies—the US resupplying Israel, the Soviet Union resupplying Egypt and Syria.

The United States, too, paid a price for its role in the war. Any American alive and conscious in 1973 will remember the oil embargo, imposed by the Arab nations in OPEC. (It would be hard to forget the lines that stretched for blocks at gas pumps, since the embargo stretched on for half a year). King Faisal of Saudi Arabia led the embargo—though, assassinated by his nephew in 1975, the Saudi king didn't survive the embargo by much more than a year. His assassin, Faisal bin Musaid, had recently returned from the US upon the death of his own father, Prince Khalid bin Musaid. The Prince—King Faisal's brother—had himself been killed during a protest opposing the King's secularizing policies. Purportedly, Musaid acted to avenge his father's murder, but I was taught that the CIA aided in the assassination.

The war went well at first for Egypt and Syria, but reversals came soon enough. Within a week, Israeli artillery shells were falling on the outskirts of Damascus. And, by the second week, the Egyptian forces had been pushed

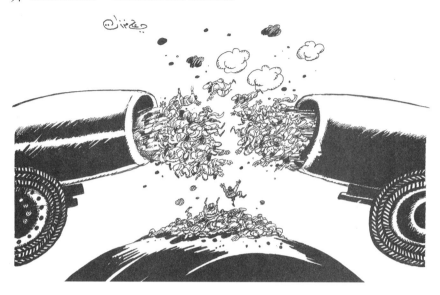

back, yielding Sinai once again. Israeli forces had completely encircled one of Egypt's three main armies and were threatening to push on to Cairo itself.

Seeing the forces of its allies in shambles, the Soviet Union pressed the UN for a cease-fire. The OPEC oil embargo was hitting the American economy, and both sides in the military conflict were suffering heavy casualties. In a little less than three weeks' time, all parties had endured enough. When the cease-fire lines were being drawn on maps of the Middle East, Egypt stood to gain somewhat, but Syria got next to nothing.

In the peace settlement of 1974, Quneitra was returned to Syria. An old Ottoman settlement, Quneitra once enjoyed a population of 20,000. But, strategically situated in the southwestern valley of the Golan Heights, it became prime real estate for Israeli occupation—which it endured for the six years between wars. Quneitra was retaken, albeit briefly, during the early days of the Yom Kippur War. It remained in Israeli hands for another six months, while peace terms were being negotiated.

When Quneitra was at last returned to Syria, there was nothing left. So the government used this war-ruined town to solicit donations from the Gulf States. As I've noted, my father worked for the Syrian Ministry of Economics and Trade, so he accompanied several foreign delegations in visits to Quneitra. In fact, the town was never rebuilt—none of it. A 2004 government census listed its population as 153. From 20,000 down to 153. I visited the site myself in 2003. It remained in waste and ruin, as if frozen in wartime. And yet, looking across the border from Quneitra into Israel, I saw a land green and lush, busy and prosperous. It was the difference between night and day.

I once saw a TV documentary about the Golan Heights and how the land prospered while under Israeli occupation. And now, I've come to understand that Assad—first the father, and then the son—made a deliberate decision to leave Quneitra a ghost-town ruin. The ruin is meant, I suppose, to serve as a visual reminder of the Israeli destruction. To me, it's a visual reminder of the hypocrisy and inefficiency of Assad's Syria.

Earlier this summer, I had a conversation with an American friend about Pyrrhic victories in war. That's when the price paid by the self-declared winner is so steep as to make any claims of victory ring hollow. Considering the loss of life and the economic devastation, Egypt and Syria paid an enormous price for the land returned. The title of O'Ballance's book, *No Victor, No Vanquished*, is spot-on. The Yom Kippur War was fought to a draw.

But the bloody battlefield draw, however Pyrrhic, proved a victory of sorts for the collective Arab psyche. After the 1967 war, the Arab states felt powerless against Israeli military might. More than demoralizing, this collective humiliation was paralyzing. But the Yom Kippur War gave the combined Egyptian-Syrian forces several days of battlefield dominance, demonstrating that their military could hold their own for more than a week against Israeli firepower, that the gap in military technology had narrowed, and that the Israeli military could no longer stand behind an aura of invincibility. Before the Yom Kippur War, the Israeli government had little incentive to pursue UN Security Council Resolution 242.

Passed in November, 1967—just months after the Six-Day War—Resolution 242 outlined the principle of "land for peace." It's arguable that October 1973 put Egypt and Israel on a path toward the US-brokered Camp David Accords. It was, indeed, a "land for peace" deal. Israel would give back the Sinai, and Egypt would make peace with Israel. It was a remarkable moment in September, 1978, when Egyptian President Anwar El Sadat shook hands with Israeli Prime Minister Menachim Begin. Later that year, these one-time "forever foes" shared the Nobel Peace Prize.

In no way should this last observation be taken as justification for the Yom Kippur War—or for any war, for that matter. No war is worth the price. If peace comes at the end of war, I welcome the peace but deplore the war nonetheless. I am no longer the eight-year-old Tarif jumping for joy as shells rain down outside Damascus and the electricity shuts off. And, truth to tell, the thirteen-year-old Tarif loathed the moment when Sadat shook Begin's hand.

At the time of the Camp David Accords, it seemed as if our old ally was selling Syria down the river. The Egyptians were getting the Sinai back, but what about the Golan Heights? (Sadat signed the peace treaty *for Egypt*. But what about the land lost elsewhere? Shouldn't the Golan have been part of any peace deal?) It's curious that a thirteen-year-old Syrian couldn't yet understand that "land for peace" entailed *peace*. President Assad would have had to shake Prime Minister Begin's hand, too. But that would never happen.

History now tells us that the Egyptians feared that including Syria in the negotiations would have weakened their bargaining position. They thought that the negotiations might collapse with no progress to show for the effort. Under these circumstances, I suppose you could say that one step toward peace was preferable to nothing, but nearly fifty years after the 1967 war, the Golan still has not been returned.

I did not mourn Sadat's death. I was sixteen years old on October 6, 1981, when he was assassinated. The Egyptian Islamists who plotted against him hated his handshake on behalf of peace, and he paid for it with his life. Sadat would be replaced by his Vice President, Muhammad Hosni El Sayed Mubarak, who ruled Egypt from 1981 to 2011—by which time, the "Arab Spring" had taken hold and spread across North Africa, bringing down heads of state in Tunisia and Libya as well as in Egypt. Crossing the Suez Canal and heading eastward, this same "Arab Spring" reached Syria in January, 2011. By February, 2012, the Syrian popular uprising had grown into a full-blown civil war and it seemed a mere matter of time before Bashar al-Assad, too, would fall.

But Bashar al-Assad did something that no other Arab strongman—not the Egyptian Mubarek, not the Tunisian Ben Ali, not even the Libyan Muammar Ghadafi—had dared in the struggle to maintain power. Pursuing a scorched-earth policy against the Syrian Free Army's urban advances, Assad began barrel-bombing his own civilian populations.

* * *

For an Islamic ethicist like myself, the Middle East today presents a gloomy picture. The rise of ISIS has merely complicated an already maddeningly complex field of religious, ethnic, political, and military conflict. The US has supported Israel, right or wrong, for sixty-five years. The Russians have supported Syria, right or wrong, for almost as long. Though the collapse of the Soviet Union reduced Russian influence during the First Gulf War of 1990-1991 (Operation Desert Storm, as it was named in the US) and the Second Gulf War of 2003, the Russian Federation under Vladimir Putin has sought to restore some of the old Soviet Union's regional clout. Consider Russia's increasingly fierce support of its Syrian ally, Assad.

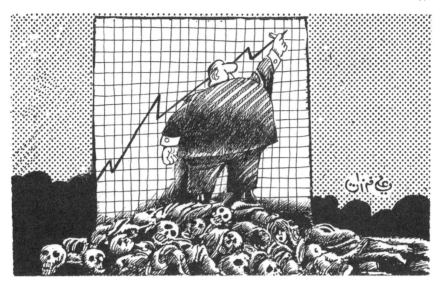

Saddest of all is the fact that war turns a hefty profit, making some people rich. I've asked myself: Why was Mr Azem doing business with Rafiq al-Natsheh? And how did Mr Azem make his fortune? An American friend told me of an old comic strip character, Little Orphan Annie, the ward of her rich benefactor, "Daddy" Warbucks. As the name implies, "Daddy" Warbucks made his money supplying the war effort—in his case, World War I. But when has it ever been different? Consider the plight of Palestinians today. For every building destroyed by an Israeli bomb, missile, or bull dozer, someone has to clean up the mess. So *someone* on the Palestinian side is going to get a contract and *someone* is going make a buck. This is true in Syria today, in Iraq, in Afghanistan.

I wish that my personal experience of war came to a close with this chapter, to be thus relegated to the imperfect memories and naiveté of an eight-year-old or thirteen-year-old or sixteen-year-old Damascene. Unfortunately, I have lived my entire conscious life with conflict raging somewhere in the Middle East, occasionally reaching to my doorstep. I would have hoped that sheer war-weariness had, by now, brought the region's opposing forces to the peace table. But such is not the case. So, while my childhood comes to a close here, the theme of war carries on into the chapters of my adulthood.

3
Endless Study, Endless War
(My First Sight of Bashar)

I came to the Prophet [peace be upon him] while he was reciting:
"Rivalry for worldly gain distracts you." He said: "The son of
Adam says: 'My wealth, my wealth.'" He said: "O son of Adam:
What is there for you out of your wealth except that which you
have eaten and wasted, or what you wore and wore out, or what
you gave in charity and it has been saved for you with God?"

—Hikam, Abd Allah ibn Shihaya

By the time I was fourteen, my mother had established herself as an independent businesswoman trading Turkish goods in Damascus. One day she
said to my brother, Samer, and me, "Let's go downtown—I have a surprise I
think you'll like!" She brought us to a big department store where we each got
to pick out a bicycle of our very own. Mine was a dazzling pink with shiny
chrome trim. I don't remember being so excited in my entire life.

My enthusiasm was dampened when we got home, however, and I realized
that bike-riding was not a native talent. At my age, I was embarrassed that
I couldn't ride, so I started practicing on our narrow balcony. Despite the
railing, it seemed precarious. It was certainly awkward. When I could stay
upright for more than a few seconds at a time, I took my practicing down to
the streets.

Soon I was riding up and down the streets near our house and past where
the Assad family was living. The Presidential Palace hadn't yet been built, so
the Assads lived in a walled villa on an affluent street in an affluent part of
the neighborhood nearby. This was in 1976, several years before the Syrian
Muslim Brotherhood began its attacks in Aleppo. This was before mere membership in the Brotherhood was declared a capital offense, before President
Hafez al-Assad's brother, Rifaat, vowed to eliminate the Brotherhood whatever the cost in blood. In his Stalinist purge of the entire nation, mere suspicion would suffice, and ten innocents would suffer for every Brother imprisoned or executed. This was before the Brotherhood's final stand in the city of

Hama in 1982, before Rifaat led the military assault that flattened the city, massacring tens of thousands.

It would be more than a decade before the New Shaab presidential palace was completed. In 1990, when the billion-dollar "People's Palace" was at last ready, Hafez al-Assad withdrew his family behind its fortress-like walls.

It's hard to imagine that there was ever a time when the Assads lived in a "neighborly" sort of way, though things would change soon enough. In the mid-1970s, there were sentry boxes by the front gate of the president's villa and, of course, there were security guards all around, but there were no military checkpoints on the streets for cars—or bicycles—to pass through. In fact, during one of my early trial-runs, I crashed near the front gate and one of the guards came out to help brush me off and get me back on my bike.

And I remember riding past a teenager about my own age who lived in this gated villa. He seemed a bit like me. Unlike the typical Syrian Arab, we both had light colored hair. (In time my hair would darken—and so would his, to Syrian black.) And we were both awkward on the road, I on my bicycle and he on his magnificent motor scooter. In my mind's eye I can see him now, a gawky teenager swerving about on his scooter. I can see his face clearly but can hardly describe the expression, which seemed sad and day-dreamy—a sort of lost look, if that makes sense. When our eyes met, his did not show the hauteur that I had come to associate with the children of Ba'athist officials. Those kids I hated to the point of scorn, but this neighborhood kid seemed unassuming, despite his villa-home and spectacular motor scooter. We didn't speak. I'm not sure if we exchanged nods. I pedaled and he sputtered off. We went our separate ways.

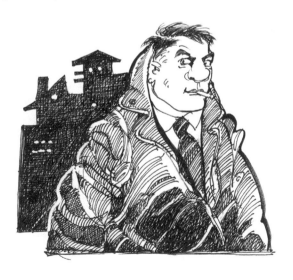

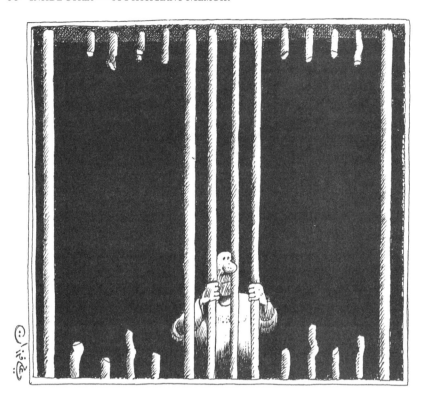

Soon enough, the neighborhood's level of security changed horribly for the worse. The Syrian Muslim Brotherhood was raising Ba'athist paranoia to a fever pitch. And, for a time, the Brotherhood was a force to be reckoned with. It led demonstrations nationwide, in the north especially. The government response, in particular the 1982 siege of Hama, was a practice-run for future government policy. Special militias and whole army units would arrive to "pacify" demonstrators, wiping out entire neighborhoods and whole towns. The siege and massacre at Hama was an example, not simply of Ba'athist brutality but of efficiency in pursuing its Stalinesque tactics.

Back in 1979, the Syrian Muslim Brothers weren't the wild-eyed radicals of ISIS and al-Qaeda. They were often intellectuals and, by today's standards, religious moderates—university students, schoolteachers, professors, professionals. In his *History of Syria*,[7] M. Clement Hall quotes from a Brotherhood leaflet: "We reject all forms of despotism, out of respect for the very principles of Islam, and we don't demand the fall of Pharaoh so that another one can take his place. Religion is not imposed by force."

The Ba'athists understood well enough that the Syrian Muslim Brotherhood represented, not a group of politico-religious agitators merely, but a political idea—a competing (and contagious) ideology that spread virally, as it were, through human intellectual contact. The Ba'athists could flatten whole neighborhoods, but it took only one survivor to pass on the "germ" of free thinking. This infectious, anti-Ba'athist "germ" needed to be quarantined. The agents of quarantine would be members of the Syrian Intelligence with the Syrian army standing behind them, and the place of quarantine would be a Syrian prison cell with the graveyard beyond.

The nation's youth were particularly susceptible to this "germ." Classmates of mine at Al-Thaqafi began to disappear. At the time, I didn't know why. It would take years, decades even, to find out why, since they were held in secret and without trial on mere suspicion of having had contact with the Brotherhood. Once, a friend of mine went to the home of a classmate who had gone missing. We didn't know what had happened and so he checked up on him. When he rang the friend's doorbell, Ba'athist agents pulled him inside and beat him ferociously. And they told him to keep his mouth shut about the beating and about his friend, because if he talked, they'd kill his family.

It took twenty years for my friend to tell us what happened and fifteen for our classmate to be released. Upon releasing my classmate, his jailors said that they had found nothing against him. *Why, then, was he jailed for fifteen years?*

Let's say that a schoolteacher gave you private lessons in math or in Arabic grammar and that this teacher was imprisoned, accused of being a member of the Muslim Brotherhood. This teacher would have been among the 30,000 suspected members that the government admitted in 2006 to having thrown in jail.[8] What the government didn't admit to was that its agents would go through the teacher's address book and spy on his personal contacts, throwing them into jail, as well.

These were frightening times in our neighborhood and home, just worrying about what catastrophe could happen at any moment, without warning, to any one of us. My father told Samer and me to stop going to the mosque on Fridays. Instead, we'd pray at home, where we'd have no chance of contact with anyone in the Brotherhood and we wouldn't go missing.

While in the US (having completed med school), I read about the Soviet KGB and the East German *Stasi*. Though these were the acknowledged masters at kidnapping and political extortion, I began to realize where the *mukhabarat*—the Syrian Military Intelligence Directorate (and other agencies

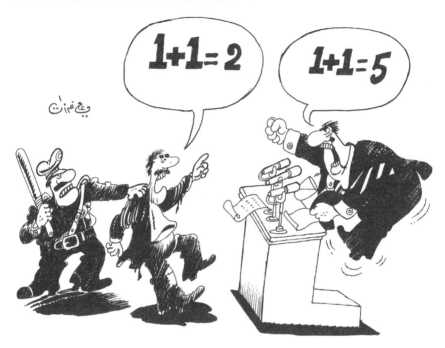

like it)—had learned their trade. And the extent of the *mukhabarat* is staggering, both in its numbers and its cost. In *Syria: The Fall of the House of Assad*,[9] David W. Lesch gives the figures:

> . . . there are estimated to be 50,000-70,000 full-time security officers in the various security branches, in addition to hundreds of thousands of part-time personnel. By 2011 there was one intelligence officer for roughly 240 people. Funding for the security services, estimated at over $3 billion per year, traditionally has made up over a third of Syria's military budget. (65)

Then as now, no one outside of the highest circles has been exempt. A lieutenant, say, in the Syrian Air Force Intelligence Directorate, or the General Security Directorate, or the Military Intelligence Directorate, or the National Security Bureau of the Socialist Ba'ath Party-Syria Region, or the Political Security Directorate could have an army general, or city mayor, or university chancellor thrown in jail "on suspicion." In other words, arrested just on his orders alone.

And there's a "James Bond syndrome" among intelligence agents. It's like they have a "double 0" license, as in "Agent Bond 007," that is. A license to kill. And they will kill you on the spot, if they feel like it. They can come to your door unannounced, break the door down, and kill you or anyone in your family. This is increasingly the scenario now, during the current troubles. But it was already the case during my teenage years. So much for my carefree youth.

* * *

Despite my family's fears and the pervasive paranoia of daily life, my school years at Al-Thaqafi might outwardly have seemed boring. Study, eat, study, eat, study, eat, study . . . sleep. But I was driven by a competitive spirit, so they weren't boring to me. I wanted to be listed, year after year, on the large bulletin board just inside the entrance doors of Al-Thaqafi as the top student in my class. I wanted to stand with the principal at a podium and receive that annual pen of achievement in front of a thousand other students. It was a cheap pen, probably made in the Eastern Bloc. But it was gold to me. And it didn't matter all that much that I didn't have many friends. I was too busy studying. (But who would have wanted me as a friend? The Tarif that I've become would find the Tarif that I was—competitive and driven to the point of obsession—insufferable.)

As I reflect back on my school years, I find that this single-minded obsessiveness made me more like a Ba'athist than I'd want to admit. It's no wonder that pride is called a "deadly sin." It blinds you to the rest of life. At least my own obsession focused on learning. But, having grown up and become an ethicist, it's clear to me that the sort of competition that requires one student winner and 999 student losers can't possibly be healthy. No wonder I had few good friends.

If, as a teenager, I had not yet learned why, I had at least learned how to study. So when I was at last humbled and my eyes opened to the Quran of peace, I had become a more spacious vessel for the lessons of God and the wisdom of the ages. As an adult, I own a collection of medals that do matter—medals of the sort given to Gandhi, Einstein, and Martin Luther King, Jr. These are more precious possessions than any cheap medal ever pinned to my chest.

Still, on one auspicious occasion, I was honored by a North Korean delegate visiting Syria. He came up to me and pinned a small medal on the chest of my dark khaki, military-style school uniform. It was a flag of Communist North Korea—bright red and blue with a red star encircled in the center. I thought my own uniform looked pretty spiffy next to the North Korean delegate's Mao-style fatigues. There were many students in attendance that day. A thousand in Al-Thaqafi's three middle school grades and a thousand in the high school grades, and we all wore the same uniform—except that mine now sported the flag of North Korea.

Syria's public schools were built on a Soviet socialist model stressing uniformity—in clothing as in curriculum. We were dressed like little soldiers, though the uniforms weren't free. Our parents paid for the government-issue uniforms, including those cheap, clunky boots that weren't fit for human wearing. I remember too well that day in the eighth grade, when my ill-fitting boots conspired with gravity and I fell, breaking my arm.

Though Al-Thaqafi School was one of the best in Damascus (indeed, in all of Syria), the curriculum was no different from any other secondary school in a nation of socialist uniformity: math, science, literature in Arabic, a foreign language (mine was English), art, music, religion (with Christians attending one class, Muslims another), and "national education." There were no private schools as in America and other Western nations. All children, even those of the highest ranking officials—even, indeed, of Hafez al-Assad, himself—endured the same curriculum with the same Ba'athist-approved textbooks in a thoroughly government-controlled school system. From school to school, the only differences would be in the quality of the teachers and the age of the facilities.

I enjoyed all my subjects, except for math—and national education. Year-in and year-out, it was the same boring lectures on the glorious achievements of the Syrian Socialist Ba'ath Party and the edifying sayings of "Our Eternal Leader, Hafez al-Assad," the "father of our country."

I shared an early draft of this chapter with an American colleague who grew up in the 1960s, during the Cold War. "What you're calling 'national education' we used to call 'civics,'" he said, adding, "the only course you took that wasn't taught in my public school was religion. My brothers and I had to go after school to church catechism class for that. So I don't see what's so different between your school curriculum and mine."

We talked a bit more, comparing notes. "There's a difference," I told him, "between pledging allegiance to the flag of one's country and pledging allegiance to a political party and its dictator." He got the message. Still, our conversation led me to realize that, despite the Ba'athist propaganda, the school curriculum of my generation was more progressive, and certainly more "secular," than curricula in many Arab countries currently. Art and music, for example, are as good as gone in Syrian classrooms today—that is, where public classes are still being held. Ironically, it was my teachers in those very subjects that left a lasting impression.

Mr Dadoush was unlike the other teachers at Al-Thaqafi. He had long hair—definitely Bohemian-*artiste* in appearance. And he was most unlike his colleagues in another respect, in that he was madly in love with his subject— music appreciation. He "made" us listen to Western classical music, which, to me, was an irresistible siren song. I loved classical music back then and still do. Chopin's *Nocturnes* were my favorite, but I loved anything by Bach, Mozart, and Beethoven. I remember hearing Beethoven's *Fifth Symphony* for the first time and almost levitating out of my seat.

As an adult, I've tried to share my love of music with fellow Syrians. In 2007, I was Director of Services for AAMAL, a nonprofit clinic serving disabled children in Damascus. The clinic had a wonderful theatre/auditorium, custom-made for medical lectures and staff meetings. "*Why not use it for culture, too?*" I thought to myself. I had fallen in love with the BBC TV program, *Classical Destinations*, which played classical music while giving visual tours of the cities and country landscapes where the great composers wrote and performed. So I reserved the auditorium and announced a public showing of the program and drew a whopping crowd of three, myself included. Though the medical specialists under me often lingered around my office, not to talk, but to listen to the music playing softly in the background.

But not all my teachers were like Mr Dadoush. Here, too, my American colleague is quick to tell stories of "the good, the bad, and the indifferent" teachers he's had over the years—but none of *his* teachers were lieutenants in the Syrian military or members of the Syrian Socialist Ba'ath Party. ("*Touché.* Most true," admits my friend, "but a couple of them might as well have been.") So now, how do I explain my seventh-grade folly when I posed the following question to my father? We were sitting together as a family, eating supper:

"Hey, Dad, what if I joined the Ba'ath Party?"

It was 1977 and I was hurling headlong toward my thirteenth birthday. I'd already lived long enough to know that Ba'athists behaved differently and were treated differently than the "mere" Syrians around me—which included my father and other family members. My father was working for the Syrian government at the time, yet he never joined the party. None of my close friends were card-carrying members of the Syrian Socialist Ba'ath Party. Neither, to my knowledge, were their parents. Outside of servicemen, I knew few Ba'athists personally. And those national education courses were boring. Why, then, would I even broach the subject?

"Well, what if I joined?"

I repeated my question, since my father hadn't given an answer. Instead, he

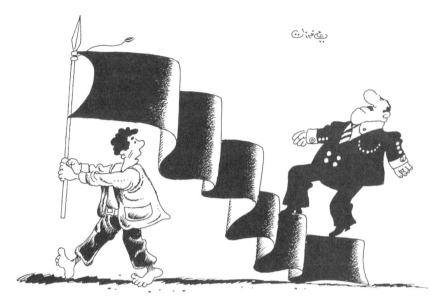

swallowed his bite of food and, picking up his water glass, took a long, slow sip. My mother stopped eating and was staring down at her plate. My older brother Samer sat back in his chair and grinned, as if settling in to watch a sitcom on TV. As I write, I wonder now if Samer had once asked this same question and already "knew the script."

Setting down his glass, my father turned toward me and, with a look of utter incredulity, replied: "Why would you want to join *them*?"

I don't remember much of the conversation that ensued. I know that my father wasn't happy. But his final words on the subject were a simple, "Do what you want."

I admire my father for that answer, though he knew I'd regret my decision. He knew there was danger in the decision, too. But he wasn't going to hold me back. He didn't hold my mother back when she asked for the virtually un-heard-of freedom to start her own business—she, a married Muslim woman in a male-dominated world. He was going to give me a similar freedom, and I was going to learn from my decision.

The Al-Thaqafi School Section of the Syrian Socialist Ba'ath Party held weekly after-school meetings in one of several special meeting rooms reserved for party use. Meetings were a rather somber affair, led by one of the school's principals who was backed up by the faculty's Ba'ath Party head. I should ob-serve that each secondary school had an army officer assigned to it. (Whether this was true in the smaller towns and villages, I can't say. But it was true in Damascus.) And every school had a faculty member—typically the teacher of national education—who served as the faculty's Ba'ath Party head. (This, I suspect, was true throughout Syria.) The faculty at Al-Thaqafi were encouraged and, I assume, pressured to join, though I didn't see any of my favorite teachers in attendance. The weekly agenda was pretty much a repetition of the national education curriculum, only there were faculty, staff, and students from different classes actually listening to the principal's lecture about the glorious achievements of the party.

After I had handed in the paperwork and took a seat, I assumed that I'd at last learn the truth about Ba'athism. As I've noted in a previous chapter, the principle of socialism—of an equitable distribution of wealth and resources—appealed to my youthful idealism. But I had questions. After my first meeting ended, I turned to an adult whom I recognized as a schoolteacher, though I had never taken a class from him.

"So, why do we stand in line to get bread and the kids of party leaders don't? Why do the kids of party leaders drive around in fancy cars and we don't?" The directness of my questions seemed to catch him off guard.

"Doesn't your father belong to the Party?" was his response: "Ask *him* why or why not." Yes, my questions were naïve. But even a child of thirteen knows when an adult gives a non-answer to a naïve question. It's not that I was seeking special treatment for myself—which might have justified a person's joining the Ba'ath Party to begin with. I simply didn't understand why, in a nation committed to socialism, there were some people treated "more equal" than others. It irked me that party members could skip to the front of any line. Unlike the rest of us, they didn't have to wait for food, for a movie ticket, or for any of the bureaucratic stamps required on the documents that were required in daily life. (So far as I could tell, members of the Syrian Intelligence didn't even need those stamps.)

So, after a few weeks of meetings, I asked the head of the Al-Thaqafi School Section of the Syrian Socialist Ba'ath Party for permission to leave. Like my father, he turned to face me, incredulous. But, unlike my father, he burst out in a fury.

"Do you *realize* how *serious* it is to *leave* the *Ba'ath Party?*" he asked, giving weight to his words. Here I was, the top of my class, one of the stars of Al-Thaqafi School—and I was asking to leave the Ba'ath Party. The audacity! Unprecedented.

The irregularity of my request was such that a committee was convened to interrogate me as to why I was leaving. My interrogators would include the army lieutenant, the faculty Ba'ath Party head, and the regional head of the party in our school district.

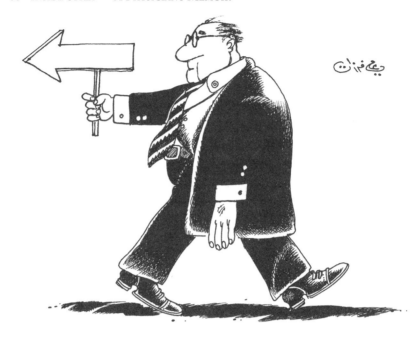

The whole school heard of the proceedings. Before the inquiry, I was pulled aside by Mr Zaeem, another teacher of mine who worried for my safety. He had crafted an excuse for me—perhaps the only one that would have worked—and he coached me ahead of the meeting. I really didn't realize the freedom- and life-threatening danger I had put myself in. I didn't realize the implications for my family, either. After all, I wasn't just dropping out of the seventh-grade Science Club!

The interrogation was held in one of the school's special meeting rooms. Each inquisitor took his turn grilling me. I had never been much of an actor, but mine was a command performance. With a choked voice and, seeming on the verge of tears, I began: "Mm . . . my . . . mother . . . is sick . . . she's so ill—she's throwing up . . . she's in terrible . . . pain. I'm afraid she'll die—she needs my help after school, every day."

My performance caught them off guard—for a moment. Then they got furious. I'd never seen grown men so angry, even hysterical. "*No one* casually quits the *Ba'ath Party*—the *sole path* to *freedom* and *power* for the *Arab people!* And *no* snot-nosed seventh-grader *ever* quits the *Ba'ath Party!*" They were out of their chairs now, looming over me as they spoke. Then they pulled me up out of my chair, set me down by the door and shoved me out: "Presumptuous ingrate! Get out of here! Good riddance!"

***

Part of "national education" was meant to prepare us for our next war with Israel, whenever that might come. I've mentioned the military uniforms we had to wear. All we lacked, seemingly, was a weapon to sling over our shoulders. So, in the ninth grade, our "class trip" was to an army rifle range. They bused us out to the countryside and handed each of us scrawny kids a heavy old Czech-supplied bolt-action rifle. Searching the web for photos, I think these may have been army-surplus Vz. 24 rifles, World War II leftovers that had possibly been used in *al-Nakba* ("The Catastrophe" in Arabic, which was how we referred to the Palestine War of 1948). It was *al-Nakba* that brought British Mandatory Palestine to an end, the nation of Israel into being, and and the horrific loss of life and land for Palestinians, an estimated 700,000 of whom were internally displaced or expelled. Many Palestinian families are still living in refugee camps such as those in Jordan, Syria, and Lebanon. They often lack documents that will allow them to travel freely or are blocked from returning to visit relatives in what is now Israel. Nearly seventy years since *al-Nakba,* the Palestinian-Israeli conflict seems endless and is still exceptionally bitter.

As a teenager, awkwardly cradling the old rifle, I didn't reflect much on its history. The regular army wouldn't trust us fourteen- and fifteen-year-olds with their precious Kalashnikovs (AK-47 assault rifles)—and I wouldn't have trusted us, either. But the Vz. 24 was a real rifle nonetheless and we were given real bullets to fire. The weapon was so heavy I could barely lift it to my shoulder. Virtually all of us missed every target every time. Part of our job was to collect the spent cartridges. So, as the boy next to me finished shooting at the targets, I saw a shell casing roll forward and began trotting after it. Thank goodness the army supervisor was watching. Violently—and luckily for me—he jerked me back by the neck of my military jacket. There were others still shooting, so I was within a split second of being the only target any kid actually hit.

I've written that my daily routine was to study, eat, study, eat, sleep. That's an exaggeration. When school was over, there was precious time for sports and games. Samer had his friends, and I had a few of my own in the neighborhood, where we'd play soccer. Of course we had no soccer field or playground. We'd just gather in the least-busy street, set two rocks (for goals) on either end, choose sides, and start kicking. I was terrible at soccer. I knew it and everyone else in the neighborhood knew it, but we were always a kid or two (or three) shy of a team and I'd give it my all. We didn't always have a soccer ball, so we'd make do. Sometimes we'd make a "short field" and kick around a Coca-Cola bottle cap.

As long as we didn't break anything or cause any trouble, the adults left us to our own devices. While there were no public playgrounds in the area, there was a recreation center where kids could play basketball and table tennis. My brother and I visited at times. Although the rec center was run by the government, the directors and the training staff were members of the Muslim Brotherhood. The Brotherhood was outlawed, so the affiliation of the staff was on the low down. Looking back, it's likely Syrian Intelligence agents were keeping tabs on the club, and it's lucky that I was not whisked away one day "on suspicion."

For there's no doubt that the Muslim Brotherhood used community centers of this sort for recruitment. That's how groups like the Muslim Brotherhood insinuated themselves into a community. They provided services that government neglects. They gained the respect of their neighbors. They placed the community in their debt, and then they began the process of indoctrination. Such was life in Assad's Syria. I could have been arrested for playing table tennis in a rec center.

You'll notice that I've been writing about my teenage years but haven't mentioned girls. There's good reason for that. There were no girls at Al-Thaqafi School. (Most Syrian schools were, and still are, segregated by gender.) I was eleven when puberty struck. It's odd how hormones work like eyeglasses. Suddenly a new world—one inhabited by girls—comes into focus. It was there all along, you just couldn't see it. Sex was not a school subject and it wasn't something that my parents talked about, so I was left to puzzle out my own feelings and changes. I started reading a Syrian magazine, *Tabebak* (meaning "Your Doctor" in Arabic), so I could understand what was happening to me. (I guess you could say that my medical studies began at this time.)

It's not that my parents were prudish or stridently religious. It's that Arab Islamic culture forbids sex before marriage, and parents back then weren't into "the birds and the bees" talk with their kids. Parents, *not* their children, decided when it was time for marriage, and it was the mother's task to find her sons suitable mates. There was no "dating" in the modern American sense of that term. Never in high school or college did I "go out on a date." While attending Damascus University—which was (Hallelujah!) coed in its student body—I did go out for coffee with groups of students, male and female together. And I enjoyed my share of small-talk, occasionally flirtatious, with female classmates. I can't lie. I loved being among college coeds. But never at the expense of modesty.

So, returning to my teenage years: I'd say, "Hi" and share a few shy words with girls in my apartment building and in the neighborhood, and my family sometimes visited the homes of other families that had daughters. That was the extent of my casual contact with women my age. When I did marry at twenty-four years old (a marriage that was ill-fated and brief), it was done with a mind toward tradition.

For my generation of Syrians, the question of marriage was a marker that divided tradition from modernity. My first wife and I were caught at a moment of transition. There were two questions on marriage: choice and approval. Who made the initial pairing? And who approved the match?

In our case, my future wife and I met when I was at medical school in Damascus and she was studying business. We met on our own—apart from the agency of our families—and this was a modern wrinkle on tradition. Still, I needed to ask the blessing of my parents and her parents—and this was serious. We would never have defied the wishes of our parents.

One of my American colleagues (who read this chapter in draft) laughed at this. "So, you let your mother choose your first wife?" he asked, teasingly.

"No, no," I replied. "My mother was used to having her own way in life, and she wasn't going to interfere with mine. Of course, my parents' marriage was arranged in the traditional manner. And they've been together for more than a half-century."

I have one last story to tell of my teenage years, and it's about my first paying job. I was seventeen and just starting eleventh grade. And I was looking forward to the Damascus International Fair (DIF), held yearly in September. Ba'athist Syria was hardly an international tourist attraction, so the Fair was my once-yearly chance to meet foreigners and get a glimpse into the way people lived elsewhere in the world.

There was a hierarchy among exhibits, now that I think about it. The second-largest was the Soviet Union's, since they were Syria's patron and institutional/bureaucratic model. The largest was Syria's own. The latest in home-grown science, technology, and manufacture was on proud display in its exhibits, all pointing to the utopian future of our nation—indeed, of our world—under Ba'athist socialism. Exhibits by Eastern Bloc countries (East Germany, Czechoslovakia, Yugoslavia, etc.) were also roomy, as were the exhibits by other Arab states. But I already knew what all these had to offer.

The exhibits that attracted me most were from Western nations. The US, Canada, the UK, West Germany, France, Italy. Compared to the Middle Eastern and Eastern Bloc exhibits, these were modest. I wouldn't be surprised if restrictions had been placed on what and how much they showed. In fact, these were mostly displays of photographs and posters. But put yourself in my place. The Internet had yet to be invented. Syrian TV showed a politically censored slice of the world, and there weren't many Western books for library lending or for sale. Do you think the textbooks approved for use at Al-Thaqafi included photos of the Eiffel Tower, the Houses of Parliament, or the Empire State Building? Yet here they were, poster-sized, in front of me. And there were real live Germans walking about in the West German exhibit, real Italians in the Italy Exhibit, real Americans, real Canadians.

The annual Damascus International Fair was intended as a showcase for Ba'athism, but what I took away from it was quite the opposite. There really was a bright and hopeful world outside of Syria.

And now for my first job: My mother had a friend at the Qatari Embassy in Syria who got me a job working at the Qatari Exhibit of the DIF. I helped watch over the exhibit during the busy daytime and cleaned up afterwards, preparing for the next day's visitors. I'll never forget my first paycheck. Working fifteen days, I earned close to $600—about four times the rate of the Ba'athist paycheck that I received some twenty years later, while teaching at the Damascus University Medical School. As was often the case in my teenage years, my initial response was confusion. How could the Qatari government pay me, a seventeen-year-old, more money for two weeks' worth of work than my father, who worked for the Syrian government at the time, made in four months?

Of course, I was thrilled to make money like a grown-up (actually, better than most grown-ups I knew) and I hoarded it like a miser glorying in the glitter of his coins. I used some of it to buy my first medical anatomy book and managed to keep the rest saved for my first trip to the States, in 1985.

There was one other reason that I looked forward to the Damascus International Fair. The American and British exhibits gave me a chance to try out my English speaking skills. The English courses that I took at Al-Thaqafi taught me to read but not to write or speak in English. To experience English as a living language, I used to visit the American Cultural Center (ACC) in Damascus—and each year, the Fair gave me the means to test my growth. If it were not for the American Cultural Center and summer courses in English, I would not have had the skills to study, work, and eventually teach in America.

Where is the ACC today? I searched the Internet. "Damascus Closes US School and Culture Center after Border Raid," declares an article from the October 28, 2008, issue of the *New York Times*. The web-archived article is referring to the Abu Kamal raid, carried out by US Special Operations forces in Syrian territory. The American-led coalition in Iraq had grown tired of Syrian trafficking in weapons and al-Qaeda fighters. So the American forces struck, the Ba'athist government reacted, and the ACC was closed.

If the Syria-Iraq border was "porous" to terrorists back in 2008, think what it's become since the Civil War began in 2011.

* * *

Wars in the Middle East didn't take a holiday during my teenage years. In fact, wars in and around Syria have spanned the entire course of my life, with many overlapping in time and most continuing in some form or other today—with no end in sight. I've already mentioned the Six-Day War of 1967, Jordan's "Black September" expulsion of the PLO in 1970, Israel's bombing of Lebanon after Black September, and the Yom Kippur War in 1973. The Lebanese Civil War lasted from 1975 to 1990. The Israelis invaded Lebanon in 1982. The Iran-Iraq War spanned nine years, from 1980 to 1988. Iraq's invasion of Kuwait in 1990 drew the US-led coalition into the first Gulf War of 1991. In 2003, the US and UK began the Second Gulf War, with occupying forces remaining in Iraq for eight years. In 2006, Israel blasted Lebanese civilian infrastructure (including Beirut's international airport) in a thirty-four-day battle against the Hezbollah. And the civil war in Syria began in 2011. By 2013, the Islamic State was running rampant throughout war-weakened Syria and the midsection of Iraq. By the summer of 2014, the US was again involved militarily, with aerial bombing of ISIS in Iraq and Syria.

I was fifteen in 1980, when the Iran-Iraq War began. In my zeal to witness history unfolding, I got a notebook to document the war day-by-day—not realizing that the war would last almost 3,000 days. I did write a paragraph or so every day for the first few months. It was a horrid affair, fought to a stalemate, costing a million lives—half of them civilian. Of course, that's not how I saw it at the time.

I was keenly partisan. In my view, it was a war between Arabs and Persians. As a teenager, I was naïve enough to root for the Iraqis in their quest to "reclaim their rightful land" from the Iranians. Only later did I realize that the US, too, was rooting for Iraq in its war against the upstart, Ayatollah Khomeini, who had overthrown the Shah of Iran—America's one-time ally.

The US had provided the Shah with a remarkable military arsenal, including jet fighters and attack helicopters. Being so well equipped, Iran should have rolled over the Soviet-supplied Iraqis—but the Ayatollah Khomeini made the same strategic mistake as the old Soviet dictator, Joseph Stalin. For reasons of ideology (and paranoia), both had purged their militaries of some of their best-trained officers. (In Revolutionary Iran, some 12,000 officers were sacked from the army alone). When Hitler began Operation Barbarossa against Soviet Russia in 1941, Stalin's officer corps had been gutted and remained unprepared. So too with Iran in 1980, which had the hardware but not the personnel. Officers who had been imprisoned—including many under orders of execution—were released and allowed to prove their loyalty to the Ayatollah. But by the time they arrived at the front, the battle lines had hardened and the Iran-Iraq War became a war of attrition.

This war, like so many wars in the Middle East, was about oil. Or was it about regional dominance? Or was it about a tyrant's ambitions? Or was it about religion? When religion is involved, every war becomes a "holy war." The Iranians, for example, gave each soldier a key on a neck chain. If he died in battle, the key would unlock the gates of Heaven. (Indeed, the funeral of a radical Islamic "martyr" today is celebrated as a wedding feast, with the martyr sent off to Heaven to receive his promised carnal rewards—often to the chagrin of his earthly widow.)

During the war, the United States gave clandestine support to Saddam Hussein. The Sunni Gulf States, Saudi Arabia especially, also supported Hussein in his war against Shiite Iran. Toward the war's end, the Soviets also lined up behind Saddam Hussein. Apparently, the Soviets did not feel immunized against the ripple effects of the Iranian revolution, even though ninety percent of the Muslims in the Soviet satellite states in Central Asia were Sunni.

In my teenage enthusiasm for the Arab forces of Iraq against the Persian forces of Iran, I did not stop to think that Syria, Iraq's neighbor and Ba'athist rival, supported Iran in the Iran-Iraq War. (Iran continues to support the Syrian regime today.) Hussein aspired to be the new Nasser, making Iraq the dominant pan-Arab regional power. But, after all of his costly adventures and the resultant loses in Iraqi blood and treasure, his fate was more ignominious than Nasser's—he was to be captured hiding in a "spider hole" by US troops and hanged by order of an Iraqi court.

Looking back, it grieves me that the teenage Tarif could ever have supported a brutal dictator like Saddam Hussein. Then again, in many wars of the Middle East, it's inevitably one tyrant or tyrannical group squaring off against another: Saddam Hussein vs the Ayatollah Khomeini, Bashar

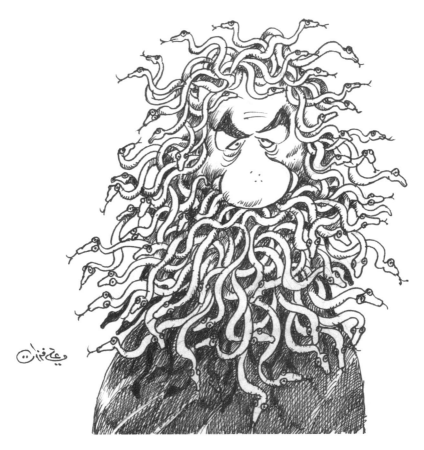

al-Assad vs ISIS. Both sides are intolerant. Both sides have committed war crimes. Typically, the "right side" is hard to identify.

As a teenager, I devoured the newspaper and magazine accounts of the Iran-Iraq War, marveling at the sheer amount of military hardware involved and the massive battles that see-sawed back and forth across the front lines. This was the largest conventional war since World War II, though it was fought a great deal like World War I (despite the modern weaponry). There were front-line trenches guarded by barbed wire and machine gun nests. The Iranians ordered massive human-wave assaults, partly to compensate for their lack of heavy weaponry. In the first waves came the poorly-trained religious volunteers, the Basij, whose bodies were used literally to clear mine fields and overrun the weakest Iraqi positions. These were followed by the better-trained Revolutionary Guards. Like the Germans in World War I, Iraq resorted to the horrors of chemical weapons, including mustard gas. It used these against the Iranians as well as their own Kurdish population, which had allied with Iran to fight Hussein's army. (Not to be outdone, the Syrian army of Bashar al-Assad has killed more of its citizens with chemical weapons than any government since Saddam Hussein's.)

Let's call the Iran-Iraq War the "Eastern Front" of my youth. The "Western Front" opened in 1982. I remember playing Atari with my friend, Nidal Kurdi, at his home. The video game was Pong, and we each had a stick controller to smash a "ball" (really a crude pixilated rectangle) relentlessly and seemingly endlessly back and forth—much like a Middle Eastern war, it occurs to me now. While playing, we heard TV news of Israel's invasion of Lebanon. Israeli forces were heading toward Beirut to destroy the PLO, once and for all.

As a people, the Palestinians have been trapped in a no-win situation for nearly seventy years. Since 1948, Palestinians have been stateless. Their leadership has been in constant search for a "host nation" and, once settled in (more or less), they've fought to influence local and national politics, seeking to gain power for themselves. Before Lebanon, it was Jordan. In 1970, the Palestinian Black September group took on King Hussein's Royal Jordanian Army and lost in its bid for power. My impulse is to criticize a recurring pattern in Palestinian politics: Palestinian leaders have overreached in seeking influence and even dominance over Arab host countries despite the fact that it's the Palestinian civilians who suffer the most. Palestinians were driven from Jordan to Lebanon in 1971, and the Israelis expelled the Palestinian leadership and militia from Lebanon in 1982. Palestinians who moved to Syria after 1948 or after Black September in 1971 were never in a position to seek power. The Assad government held them tightly in check. The Palestinian search for a home has had a strong impact on every country that borders Israel.

As I've noted, my mother's family lived in Jordan. Sadly, then, I had some cousins who supported the PLO while others supported the Jordanian army. (I couldn't have predicted this back in 1982, when I was playing Atari with Nidal, but I would marry a Palestinian refugee: my wife, Remaz, is Palestinian. Her grandparents lived in what is now Israel by Lake Tiberias, which borders on the Golan Heights. At one time, they were wealthy hotel owners. In 1948, however, they found themselves fleeing for their lives, penniless, to Syria.)

Actually, the 1982 invasion that I followed as a teenager was merely the latest twist in a civil war that had begun in 1975 and would last until 1990. Before the arrival of the Arafat's PLO, Lebanon was a functioning multi-sectarian and multi-cultural state. It had tensions, especially between Christians who had greater political power and Muslims who had greater numbers. In 1958, the factions came close to civil war. Still, many look back at this period as a time when Sunnis, Shiites, and Maronite Christians lived together in peace and prosperity. This tenuous balance was upset with the expulsion of PLO fighters from Jordan to Lebanon. The Palestinian leadership sought (once again) to assert its power locally—this time at the expense of the local Christian power structure.

It was in Beirut in 1972 that my mother received her greetings from the Mossad—an act of Israeli retaliation against Black September. By 1975, the PLO had created "a state within the state" that would effectively militarize the hundreds of thousands of Palestinians already living in southern Lebanon. With the country's delicate sectarian balance undermined, the Maronite Christians raised up militias to fight the PLO, while the PLO found allies among Sunnis, socialists, and pan-Arab Muslims. Soon, all of Lebanon was engulfed in sectarian warfare.

In 1976, Lebanese President and Maronite Christian, Suleiman Frangieh, called upon his Syrian neighbor to help restore order. The Arab League affirmed Syria's peacekeeping presence in the Bekaa Valley. For its part, Israel feared the PLO build-up and was angered by continuous cross-border attacks. By 1978, Menachim Begin had endured enough. Israeli forces were ordered to enter and occupy southern Lebanon. Before withdrawing later that year, the Israelis established a twelve-mile wide buffer zone across their southern border with Lebanon.

One of the effects of a fifteen-year-old civil war is that people become numb to the horrors. For example, the father of a family living in a high-rise apartment complex might excuse himself from the dinner table to go up to his roof and fire off a mortar at enemies in an adjacent section of Beirut. His family would hear the "thwump" of the mortar shell, the father would return, and dinner would proceed: "Pass the humus, son."

Back to 1982: The Israelis mounted a full-scale invasion of Lebanon aimed at destroying the PLO. I remember that our next-door neighbors, who were Palestinian, left Damascus to fight in Lebanon against the advancing Israeli forces. I doubt that they did much good—or even arrived in time. The Israeli military swept northward to the outskirts of Beirut and laid siege. Humiliated by the swiftness of the Israeli advance, Yasser Arafat's forces faced annihilation.

Unready for martyrdom, Arafat accepted a UN-brokered deal that sent the PLO leadership out of Lebanon and into exile in Tunisia. One can imagine the scene on loading docks in the port of Beirut, where Arafat and his crestfallen fighters lined up to board a ship bound for Tunis. During their passage into exile, they were escorted by a US warship and "protected" on shipboard by US marines.

My parents were glad to see Arafat go. As an adult, I can understand why: Arafat's brand of military resistance (and the endemic corruption within his organization) had brought only troubles upon the Palestinians—and upon the Lebanese and Jordanians and even, indeed, upon my own family. Back then, I lamented the fact that so many had died so needlessly. I had at least learned compassion for the people caught up in such senseless sectarian violence. But, as a seventeen-year-old Syrian, I believed that I had witnessed little more than another Arab defeat at the hands of the Israelis.

The Lebanese Civil War was a bloody mess from every angle. The international peacekeeping force, which included American soldiers, proved unable to keep the peace. In fact, the first recorded suicide attack against American interests came in April, 1983, when a car bomb (Iranian-sponsored) struck the US Embassy in Beirut, killing seventeen American citizens and sixty-three people in total. Later in October, an even more devastating suicide attack (again Iranian-sponsored) targeted the Beirut headquarters of US and French forces, killing 241 American and 58 French soldiers. (By that one dynamite-filled truck, more US marines died at a stroke than had died in any engagement over the previous thirty-five years.) The Americans left Lebanon to its own devices while Syria—still an occupying force—vied with Iran for influence. Though the Civil War ended officially in 1990, Lebanon has remained a mere pawn in the region's power struggles.

In war it's always the civilians who suffer the most. The elderly, the mothers, the children especially. Whether Sunni or Shia or Maronite Christian, all of Lebanon suffered atrocities. There were victims, and perpetrators, on all sides. I know that now. As a Syrian teenager, I saw media coverage of only some of these. There has always been a political bias in Syrian media, though I didn't always know that. One particular atrocity that the Syrian media covered in depth—and sadly, deservedly so—was the massacre by the Maronite Christian militia, the Phalangists, of Palestinians in two refugee camps, Sabra and Shatila. These camps were controlled by Israeli troops under the authority of Ariel Sharon who approved the entry of the Phalangists into the camps. Over the course of two nights, from the evening of September 16 to the morning of September 18, 1982, as many as 3,500 Palestinians were murdered. Most were women, children, and the elderly, since the military-aged men were off fighting with the PLO. Photographs of the aftermath of those massacres remain vivid in my memory. Such photos have become all-too-familiar now, but back then they were shockingly new to me: graphic photos of innocent civilians gunned down where they lived—literally, gunned down where they lived and worked (or played) and ate and slept. Many were gunned down in the midst of their flight. And their crumpled bodies were piled up against walls and on the sidewalks, each contributing its share to the pools of blood that spread across the dusty ground.

Different causes have been given for the massacre. At the time, some called it revenge for a political assassination. Others called it genocide—an instance of "ethnic cleansing." What struck me back then, and what strikes me now, is that the massacre could not be explained away as the temporary madness of men caught up in blood lust revenge. I say this, because the sun set and rose on the first day of their killing—and, in the cold light of that first morning, the Phalangists must surely have surveyed the scene before them. Surely they heard the cries of survivors and the moans of victims not yet dead. The killing spree must have tired them out. They must have been hungry after a night of blood lust. Some, I hope, had the conscience to ask, "*What have we just done?*" I hope that at least some few shrank back in horror at their handiwork. But what strikes me is the deliberateness with which the militiamen must have rested, took a bite to eat, and then returned to the streets for a second night of carnage.

Whether it's Muslims massacring Christians or Christians massacring Muslims doesn't matter to me now, though it mattered to me back then. Murder is murder and an offense against God. What increases my grief, even to this day, is the recognition that Israeli forces, having displaced the PLO in southern Lebanon, had become an occupying army charged with "keeping the peace." The civilians in Sabra and Shatila were under their control and, hence, under their protection.

It's not that the Israelis murdered Palestinians at Sabra and Shatila. It's that they didn't stop the murders. They stood by and watched and did nothing. Actually, that's not entirely true. I've read an account recently that said the Israelis fired flares around the camps, lighting up the nighttime sky to give Phalangists better aim at their targets. If there was ever a time and a place that the Israelis could have shown their humanity and compassion toward Palestinians, it would have been at Sabra and Shatila on the evening of September 16, 1982.

The United Nations condemned the massacre. Declaring Ariel Sharon's "personal responsibility," the Israeli government's own Kahan Commission faulted the Defense Minister for "ignoring the danger of bloodshed and revenge" and "not taking appropriate measures to prevent bloodshed." (I quote the Commission report from Ze'ev Schiff and Ehud Ya'ari's book, *Israel's*

Lebanon War.[10]) Sharon survived politically. Indeed, he was elected Israeli Prime Minister in 2001. But the shame of Sabra and Shatila led at the time to his resignation as Defense Minister. The event had ripples on the Palestinian side as well. One example concerns four Palestinian teenagers who lost friends and family in Sabra and Shatila.

Three years later, in 1985, the PLO had been exiled to Tunis and was engaged in a furious back-and-forth with Israel. Both sides hoped to score media points. Victory in the media was the only possible measure of success, since the tit-for-tat style of engagement precluded an opening for peace negotiations. Neither side could afford to be seen as backing down. In retaliation for the Mossad kidnapping of a Palestinian commander in September, the PLO captured two Mossad operatives—or were they tourists as the Israelis claimed?—and executed them. In retaliation, Israeli aircraft bombed PLO offices in a neighborhood of Tripoli, killing 50 Palestinian office workers, 215 Tunisian civilians, and wounding another 100.

Two weeks later, the PLO responded with the *Achille Lauro* hijacking. The plan was for PLO commandos to travel incognito on the Italian luxury liner to the Israeli port of Ashdod. Then they were supposed to engage Israeli forces. The four teenagers selected as operatives by the PLO, were quick to figure out that this was a suicide mission. And Italian luxury on this voyage and on a previous training mission may have widened their horizons beyond what they had known in camps such as Sabra and Shatila. When their plot was discovered (or did they invite discovery?)—they gave up on Ashdod and commandeered the ship instead. Although this might have seemed a way for "no one to get hurt," they ended up killing an American retiree in a wheelchair: Leon Klinghoffer, a Jew from a prominent New York family. The media feasted on this act of barbarism and emblazoned *Achille Lauro* in public consciousness as the mark of terror.

In 1988—when Iran and Iraq came to peace terms—I was graduating from Damascus University Medical School. In 1990—when Lebanon was declared "at peace" from its Civil War—I was already in the United States, pursuing my medical residency and continuing my studies. So, here's enough (for now) of war. In my next chapter, I'm off to med school.

4
Parachuters in Med School
(Meeting Bashar without Losing My Head)

"O Allah's Messenger! Should we seek medical treatment for our illnesses?" He replied: "Yes, you should seek medical treatment, because Allah, the Exalted, has let no disease exist without providing for its cure . . ."

—Hadith, Fiqh us-Sunnah

During the 1981-1982 school year, I, like other ambitious sixteen- and seventeen-year-old Syrians in their final year of high school, had a miserable time studying day-and-night, agonizing on the hot coals of academic anxiety, trying to master the Baccalaureate tests that, at year's end, would determine my future. I even took additional, after-school classes at Al-Thaqafi, hoping to improve my test scores.

It turns out that I did well and, like other top scorers on the tests, that meant I was headed for medical school—which would carry me up several rungs on the socioeconomic ladder. My future looked bright and my family was proud. I would be following in the footsteps my paternal uncles, Bashar and Hisham, both alumni of the Damascus University Medical School.

At the same time that I was finishing high school, President Assad's brother, General Rifaat al-Assad, was putting the finishing touches on his siege of Hama. The Muslim Brotherhood—a Sunni-Islamist export from Egypt—had turned the town into a center of anti-government protest, and the Ba'athists had endured enough. General Rifaat al-Assad's tactics were thorough. He would break the back of the Muslim Brotherhood's resistance in Syria, whatever the cost. Across the twenty-seven day siege, 1,000 Syrian soldiers and paramilitary forces died. Estimates of civilian deaths vary from 20,000 to as high as 40,000. Of course, Syrian TV told us only of the victory, not of the

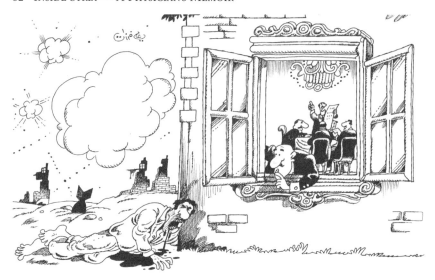

human cost. In her book, *Dreams and Shadows*, Robin Wright calls the Hama massacre one of the "deadliest acts by any Arab government against its own people in the modern Middle East."[11] We know now that Hama was a mere prelude of what was to come.

I suppose I was too busy studying back then to notice or care. Besides, the Muslim Brotherhood was a bunch of "trouble makers," right? So, the siege ended and my senior year ended and off I went to med school. In my imagination, I was entering an elite academy, handpicked out of thousands. I played out the moment in my mind when I would first greet the forty or so students who would make up my med school class. What great things we would achieve, together!

I can't express my dismay and disgust when, upon entering the school auditorium on that first day, I found myself sitting among 1,200 first-year medical students, all waiting for class to begin. I soon learned that 400 of us were the top scorers on the Baccalaureate tests while the other 800 were young Ba'athist cronies, academically unqualified, whom the rest of us took to calling Rifaat's "parachuters." So much for my dreams of a Syrian intellectual elite.

But there was an elitism at work. As a matter of politics merely, the common Syrian soldier wouldn't rush off to kill fellow citizens, putting his own life at risk. So Rifaat built his own paramilitary forces, the so-called "Defense Companies" that were loyal to him personally. They were recruited from among teenagers whose families were either Ba'ath party members or had "the right connections" among Ba'athists. Rifaat's student-recruits weren't particularly smart. But they were brutally effective in battle and they did have to pass a test of sorts to qualify for medical school.

They had to jump out of an airplane—twice I think, or maybe three times. I don't think that would qualify them as paratroopers in any Western military sense, but it did mean that they had survived a couple of plane rides and parachute jumps (which did show some loyalty and some courage on their part—I wouldn't have strapped a Soviet-made parachute on my back for any purpose under any circumstances).

Rifaat promised his hand-picked paramilitary corps that, having obeyed his orders and having passed the parachute test, they would be eligible to enroll in any Syrian school of their choice to study any discipline of their choice. And, since medical school was the most prestigious, some 800 of them were now my colleagues. So much for test scores and enrollment standards. In Assad's Syria, all you had to do was join the Ba'ath party, commit an atrocity or two, jump out of a plane, and enter medical school. If, in later chapters, I seem to exaggerate the dismal state of Syrian health care, please remember the story I've just told—and remember that many of these parachuters are "practicing medicine" today.

My disappointment was overwhelming. I had worked so hard . . . for this. I found myself sitting in the last row of a cavernous auditorium in sweltering heat with no air conditioning. The room stank from the sweat of 1,200 bodies. I tried to concentrate, but I couldn't hear and could barely see the professor standing at his podium.

I learned the routine quickly enough. Read the textbook, come to class if you feel like it, but above all, don't call attention to yourself. There were further "rules of the game." Unless you were willing to be verbally abused in public, you dared not ask a question in class. A question was like a challenge to the professor's authority. Either he was being unclear (and how could that be?) or you were being a blockhead. Also, you didn't bother to visit professors in their offices, since they weren't going to be there. And if they were, they'd wonder aloud why you had come to interrupt them, dragging them from their own more important tasks.

Since the goal was to complete med school as quickly as possible, you learned to do the minimum required. Of course, there's a difference between preparing to practice medicine and simply "getting through med school." I never became cynical about the task. I always took medicine as a high, noble

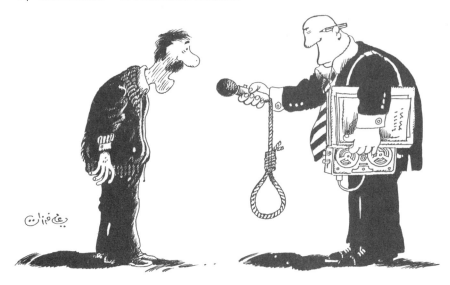

calling, despite the militant indifference of many faculty and fellow students. But I did learn to avoid courses in theory while focusing on practical subjects like anatomy, pathology, and histology.

Outside of class, I spent much of my time socializing with students from other schools in Damascus. Of course, my favorite conversation partners were the women students. Having attended an all-male high school, it was refreshing to share classes with coeds.

While the veterans of Rifaat's Defense Companies failed to distinguish themselves in the classroom, they made their presence felt in the streets of Damascus. One day, in a collective (and, I assume, planned) rampage, they walked the streets, ripping the veils off of Muslim women (and even off of Christian nuns) to protest what they called the "old thinking." It was a shocking display of disrespect, given the importance of religious observance in Syrian society. But these young Ba'athist zealots were bent on showing who was boss.

Beyond their reckless display of power, it seemed that the med-school parachuters were sending Damascenes a reminder of Hama—of how thoroughly they had routed the Muslim Brotherhood and its "troublemakers." For the first time as a Syrian, I felt the urge to ask, "What really happened there?" I asked this of students whom I felt I could trust, several having experienced the carnage close-up. Some came in time to trust me and told me what, if found out, they'd have been punished for telling.

Official Syrian media did not tell me what they, the eye-witnesses and survivors, told me. In Hama, the killing began at a distance, with rockets and heavy artillery blasting large blocks of housing into rubble, killing and maiming innocent men, women, and children indiscriminately. I'm left now with an image of shattered, shredded human bone and tissue intermingled with crumbled concrete and twisted iron rebar. Where a family once lived, splintered furniture and mangled toys remained.

After the rockets and artillery, General Rifaat al-Assad sent in the ground troops—the Defense Companies in the lead—tasked with killing teenaged males fourteen years and older. As the cruelest form of emotional torture, parents were forced to watch their boys slaughtered while they were themselves spared. I recoiled in disbelief but, over the years, I've heard this same story time and again. The Ba'athists were using Hama as an object lesson for the rest of Syria.

Had I been raised in Hama and attended school there in my senior year, I might have been among the fourteen-, fifteen-, sixteen-, and seventeen-year-old victims of Ba'athist "instruction." Having heard the stories, I thought back to my own senior year and to the fact that several new students showed up from different parts of the country, the Hama region particularly. I never thought to ask why, and I suppose it was safest that I did not. Again, it was a cold, calculated lesson to survivors: "We've killed your four older sons, but we'll send your youngest son and daughter to finish school in Damascus. Nothing personal, of course."

Early in my first semester at med school, I met an old acquaintance from elementary school, Ali Tourkmani. He was the son of Hasan Tourkmani, a prominent Ba'athist and, at the time, a Major General in the Syrian Army. Rising through the ranks, Hasan was named Minister of Defense. At the outbreak of the current civil war, he was made a member of the "team of four" charged with destroying the Free Syrian Army. Instead, the Free Syrian Army destroyed him.

Fast forward thirty years: On July 8, 2012, rebels bombed the "untouchable" National Security Building in Damascus, killing General Tourkmani, Major General Hisham Ikhtiyar (Bashar's national security advisor, specializing in "anti-terrorist" operations against the Muslim Brotherhood in Syria), and Tourkmani's Deputy Defense Minister, Assef Shawkat. In 1983, Shawkat was an officer in Rifaat's Defense Companies and an active participant in the Hama massacre. He would also become President Assad's brother-in-law. (This bombing of Syrian National Security headquarters remains, arguably, the rebel forces' boldest stroke to date. Back in July 2012, it seemed a mere matter of time before the Free Syrian Army punched its way through the barricades of my old neighborhood near Mount Qasioun to storm the

Presidential Palace. What seemed inevitable back then has become little more than a pipe dream.)

One day, Ali said to me, "Let's go eat lunch!" Since I received twenty-five dollars per month for expenses, I thought this was an inspired idea. We'd be going to al-Tai, a restaurant where I planned to gorge myself on *ful*, a favorite dish of mine made with fava beans. And there were other foods in store. Ali drove us in his BMW. As I've noted, all the children of high-ranking officials drove fancy cars—BMWs, Mazdas, and Mercedes (their favorite)—while the rest of us dreamed of someday riding in one.

I had mixed emotions while riding with Ali. The automobile was the most obvious symbol of the power that the powerful enjoyed in daily life. As a high school student, the very sight of a big car with black-tinted windows angered me. But now, cruising along with Ali in expectation of a great meal . . . somehow, it didn't seem all that bad.

As Ali drove us along, I noticed another car following us. Looking through the side mirror I saw four, maybe five big, hulking guys with huge mustaches. I knew that, tucked out of sight, their AK-47s stood at the ready.

Two other med students met us for lunch. One of them, I soon learned, was Ahmad Saleh, the son of an Air Force officer in charge of the nation's rocket program. Beyond that family connection, he didn't leave much of an impression. The other one was tall and lanky, with pleasant blue-green eyes. When we seated ourselves at the restaurant, I sat to the right of the tall guy and started joking with him and the others.

"What's your name?" I asked the tall guy.

"Bashar," he replied, in a husky baritone.

"Bashar what?" I asked, chewing on my food.

"Assad."

I felt my heart drop into my stomach. "Are you related to the . . ."

—for some reason, I pointed to the sky—

" . . . to the President?"

"Yes," he said, smiling.

My impulse was to get up and run—as fast as I could. Remember, I had just learned the uncensored truth of the Hama massacre. And, while my father had taught me to love Syria, he also taught me to hate Ba'athism. As a teenager, I had suffered my own run-ins with Ba'athism. And now, here I was, sitting at lunch with the son of the man who had sent his brother, Rifaat—Bashar's uncle—to kill tens of thousands of Syrians. I was out of my league.

I survived the rest of the lunch. Bashar al-Assad turned out to be as pleasant

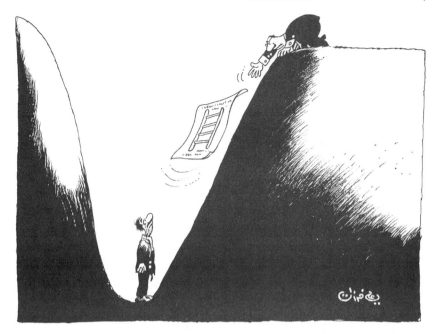

as he appeared. He laughed when, toward the end of lunch, I asked, "Did I say anything wrong?"

Occasionally afterward, I would meet Bashar at the medical school and we would chat for a few minutes. I found him to be modest and even humble, unlike most of the politicians' kids that I had known. Unlike them, he drove a modest car. He wore regular jeans, not designer jeans. He used to cover his mouth while talking, because he spoke with a slight lisp. He also had a habit of blinking overmuch while speaking. I've heard people call this a facial twitch or tick, but I wouldn't go that far. Such gestures of insecurity made me feel a little sorry for him and, yes, even like him a little bit. Though I was in no way awe-struck or inspired by him, I admit I did like him.

Some students wanted to befriend him, but many were intimidated by his status. Personally, I was neither desirous nor fearful of his company. He seemed, so far as I could tell, a serious, dedicated student—much like I was. After medical school in Damascus, he went to England to study ophthalmology. That didn't surprise me. Before being ensnared by politics, he held the rank of colonel, working as a physician in the Syrian army. Had he not become President, I've no reason to think that he wouldn't have practiced competently.

Of course, these are my personal observations. I know others from med school who remember Bashar differently. Recently, I came across an *Aljazeera* article (first published in August 6, 2012), in which fellow classmates Zaher Sahloul, Hasaan Alzein, and Maher Basatneh reminisce about their Ba'athist schoolmate.[12] I don't remember Maher, but I do remember Hasaan and I've stayed in touch with Zaher. (In fact, my friend Zaher will play a role later in this memoir.) Like me, he left Syria for the States. Currently, Dr Sahloul is teaching at the University of Illinois at Chicago College of Medicine—yet another Syrian come to America. (It turns out that his fellow *Aljazeera* interviewees all live and work in the Chicago area.)

In the article, titled "My Classmate is a War Criminal," Zaher wonders aloud how it is that Bashar al-Assad (whom he describes as "a very average and humble person") "turned out to become the architect of the ongoing bloodshed in Syria." His interview continues:

> "You never imagine that the person who used to be your classmate in medical school will be able to do this type of war crimes against humanity," said Sahloul, a native of Homs and president of the Syrian American Medical Society. . . .
>
> "He wasn't arrogant," Sahloul said. "But from what I've seen he wasn't that smart or distinguished." Sahloul recalled that two years into the presidency of his old college classmate, he and his fellow Syrian American doctors had a chance to meet Assad at a conference in Damascus. While exchanging pleasantries, Sahloul recalled Assad as saying he wished he was a practicing doctor instead of being a president.
>
> At the same meeting, Sahloul said he asked Assad if he thought Syria was ready for democracy. Assad reportedly said no, citing Syria's tribal culture and sectarian nature.

I believe it: Bashar would have chosen medicine over politics had he been given the chance. And I believe his confession-of-sorts to Zaher that democratic reform was never in his plans as Syrian President. (Had I known that, I would never have written that fateful letter to him, offering to return and teach in Damascus. . .)

In 2012, when my old med school classmate gave this interview, it seemed inevitable that the Assad regime would crumble: "Definitely the regime has ended," Sahloul said. "No one in Syria will let this regime lead anymore. People have broken the barrier of fear, so it's impossible for him to continue ruling Syria. It's not a matter of if, it's a matter of when."

But this has proved a false prophecy. As of February 2016, Assad remains in power. And Syria's health care crisis has worsened. Still, my friend's words seem carefully weighed. I can't say quite the same for Dr Alzein and Mr Basatneh, whose words present a mixture of bravado and naiveté interspersed with an occasional furtive glance at current "conditions on the ground." The interview continues:

> Like Sahloul, Alzein found Assad unremarkable. "We tried to avoid him," Alzein said. "His father was a barbaric dictator and we always said that if we get close to him, someday we will be targeted by the regime."
>
> One Chicago resident who did get close to Assad was Maher Basatneh, who is originally from Damascus. The Chicago businessman said he first befriended the future president in 1980 when they were teenagers at a skydiving camp.
>
> "He was friendly," Basatneh said of Assad. "He ate with us and we just talked as friends. He did not know anything about politics." The two became friends and would hang out at the Assad residence. There, Basatneh said, he would often witness Maher al-Assad taunt his elder brother, Bashar, calling him a "dummy."
>
> "I have known this guy for years and the position of president is not for him," said Basatneh, adding that he would not also entrust his life to Assad as his doctor. Basatneh claimed Assad was not a serious medical student, and only graduated because he was the son of the president.

Mr Basatneh—who didn't finish med school—has a perfect right to his opinions. More, he claims a closeness to the future president that made him witness of Bashar's belittling at the hands of family members. I can believe that. Again, the Assad family never expected the shy, awkward second son to replace the iron-fisted father. And this sort of abuse may well have fed an inferiority complex that Bashar, the "lion of Syria," over-compensates for by shows of strength. But I don't believe that Bashar's medical degree was mere cronyism. It's quite enough to call him a dictator. But he was not, in fact, a "dummy," and I believe he earned his medical degree. And, with all my heart, I wish that he *had* been able to stick to medicine and stay out of Syrian politics.

* * *

Returning to my own story: As a medical student at Damascus University, I did my first clinical training at al-Mouwasat Government Hospital, "the leading public hospital in Damascus." That's the subtitle of a web page describing itself as Syria's "first online museum."[13] I assume it's a government-supported website, but no matter. The web page shows a photograph, dated 1944, of the hospital's founders. A further web-search tells me that al-Mouwasat was

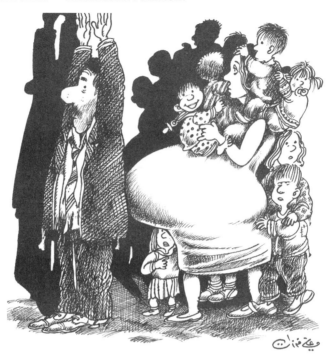

completed in 1958, and its facilities show it. (A newer facility, the Al-Assad University Hospital, was built in 1988—the year that I graduated from med school. Obviously, I never had the chance to work at Al-Assad.)

Like all public hospitals, al-Mouwasat was run by the government. There were also facilities reserved for the military, and there were some private hospitals and clinics for those who could afford them. My experience at al-Mouwasat was typical of public health care in Ba'athist Syria in the 1980s, though what I'm going to write may prove shocking to some. If I hadn't experienced it, I'd be in disbelief, myself. But I was there and I saw it, so nothing shocks me when it comes to Ba'athist Syria.

Visitors to today's American hospital floors are used to long corridors with semi-private rooms. But the ward I was assigned to was one large room holding two rows of many beds. And there were three toilet "closets" to serve the patients of the entire ward. Let me repeat that. Three toilets for all the sick patients. Actually—for reasons I shall explain shortly—there were only two toilets available. And they were always clogged.

Normally, when there's a problem like a perpetually-clogged toilet, you blame it on the laziness of housekeeping and, by extension, on the disincentive of working for peanuts in a socialist health care system. You might even assume that the problem of a clogged toilet could be solved with a bribe, which is how most work orders got prioritized by a chronically-underpaid staff. But the problem here was simply unfixable. There were too many people flushing too much waste too fast down old pipes that couldn't handle the traffic—so the toilets would be fixed for a day and stopped up for a week, fixed for a day and stopped up for a week, and so on.

The ward staff kept the third toilet under lock-and-key, for its own use. Now that's elitism. The luxury of being able to use a clean bathroom and doing so despite the suffering of patients around you. In desperation, family members brought in newspapers. In the corners of the hospital ward, they'd set the newspapers down for their sick relatives to relieve themselves—literally, they'd defecate on newspapers in the corners of the ward. Do I need mention the smell, the embarrassment, the sheer lack of hygiene entailed in this practice?

"And what about the relatives or the parents of the sick kids at the children's hospital?" you might ask. "Would they just leave, find a public toilet somewhere, and come back?" Well, that assumes that visitors could come and go as they pleased. Parents were allowed in to see their children for short times only. And, besides, when you left the hospital, where would you go if you were poor and had come from out of town? Those who couldn't afford hotels slept on the pavement outside hospital doors. In 1983, while I was in training at the children's hospital, the poorer parents were sleeping in front of its doors. And they were still sleeping in front of the Pediatric Hospital in 2010, when I left Syria for good.

A visit to any public hospital was demeaning to patients and families alike, and I blame much of that on the Ba'ath Party's Soviet-style approach to social programs. Soviet influences upon Syrian medicine and medical training were strong—and bad. Many of the professors had been trained in Eastern Bloc countries and seemed to have no clue how to treat patients humanely. Most were Ba'athists who received their appointments as rewards for party loyalty, not for competence in their disciplines. Doing the rounds with these professors was almost pointless, since there were so many students assigned to so few teachers that there was no way that we could each do a hands-on examination. Even worse, most of the teachers didn't seem to care whether we learned or not. Their attitudes toward students—as toward patients and their families—ranged from indifference to impatience to irritation to downright resentment.

Dehumanizing. That's what it was like for the patient, the patient's family, and the medical students in training. Acts of kindness and genuine concern were exceptions to the rule.

The sanitation, as I've noted, was terrible. And, compounded by a scarcity of resources, children would come sick to hospital where they would get even sicker. Three infants might share the same oxygen tent—something that would never be allowed in a Western hospital. Needless to say, if one infant had a respiratory infection, the others got it, as well.

Now, flash forward to 2009, when I had long since completed my studies and progressed in my career, having been named Secretary General for the Disabled in Syria. I was approached by the Wellcome Trust, a British non-profit organization whose educative mission includes medical humanities and the introduction of medical science into regional cultures. Under the auspices of the Wellcome Trust, I was asked to teach a course in medical communication skills. Thinking back to my own experiences as a med student, of course I said yes.

My class consisted of twenty residents training in obstetrics/gynecology at the Syrian Ministry of Health. There had been numerous, serious complaints about how women in labor were being treated. The women were being yelled at and hit. In addition to this emotional and physical abuse, their lives (and the lives of their children) were being endangered by a horrifying neglect of sanitation—women were being forced to deliver on tables still smeared with the blood and feces of women who had delivered before them.

So, I rolled up my sleeves and began talking about communication skills in medicine and the ethical treatment of women in labor. The residents listened semi-attentively for a while, until one raised his hand. "Excuse me," he began, "but how do you expect us to act 'ethically' when we're asked to work six days in a row without be allowed to go home, when our salaries are just 150 dollars a month, and when our supervisors treat us like slaves?"

His questions left me speechless. I wanted to say that none of what he had said excused hitting a pregnant woman or endangering the life of her child. But then I realized that it was futile to expect humane treatment and compassion from people who were not being treated as human beings themselves. Before I could teach the residents in training, I needed to teach ethics and communication skills to their teachers. But I suppose someone in that group would respond in much the same way: "How do you expect us to act 'ethically' when we're asked to work six days in a row, when our salaries are extremely low, and when superiors treat us like trash?" So I'd have to go up the next rung in the Ba'athist hierarchy . . . and so on, always hearing that it's always people in the chain of command above them that impose inhumane work conditions. Such is the Soviet-style approach to social programs. The person to be held responsible for a break-down in ethics or communication is never standing in the room—but he is presumed to be watching and listening.

If students from the medical school were indifferently trained, the nursing students were worse off. Syrian society has long looked down on nurses, so most nursing students came from poorer families outside of Damascus. Though they sat on the bottom rung of the Ba'athist health care system, they'd at least have a guaranteed job and room and board upon graduating.

They were taught by the same physicians that trained the med students, so they were given even less time and attention. In general, Syrian nurses could do very little, since they were taught very little. I taught nursing ethics at the School of Nursing in Damascus University from 2007 to 2010, and I believe I was the first to teach Western concepts in nursing ethics. I did what I could to improve their training, but the obstacles they faced—or that we faced, together—were institutional and endemic.

Given these problems, you'll not be surprised that people would try to treat and medicate themselves. In Syria before the recent troubles, buying drugs was easy. All you had to do was walk into a pharmacy, ask for a drug, and pay the money. The pharmacist would sell anyone anything except—maybe—narcotics. And the price of medicine in Syria was cheap compared to American pharmaceuticals. There, you could have bought ten days' worth of antibiotics for a dollar. Here, those same antibiotics would require a prescription and cost 100 US dollars or more without insurance. Of course this lack of regulation led to abuses. Laying aside the misuse of drugs in general, the over-use of antibiotics has created drug-resistant strains in Syria as throughout the world. But what was once a problem has become a crisis. The civil war has virtually destroyed the Syrian pharmaceutical industry, creating desperate shortages nationwide. It's no longer a matter of buying drugs "under the table," but of buying anything from anyone for any amount of money.

This all sounds pretty bleak, I know. But it wasn't the lack of resources, the lack of regulation, the incompetence and lack of training, the inhumane treatment, the lack of basic hygiene, or the politicizing of teacher appointments that was most offensive to me. What our Soviet mentors brought to Syrian medicine was a culture of graft that victimized family members and turned patients into exploitable commodities. For institutionalized corruption had "become a way of life" in Assad's Syria, as

David W. Lesch notes:

> . . . palms [had] to be greased for just about everything—from fixing a plumbing problem to repairing a pothole in the street. From getting a license to starting a business to obtaining a favorable judgment at court. And this way of life in Syria was exploited by the rich and powerful: if you were well connected, you got better service. (65)

To Lesch's list of palms expecting to be greased, one must add Syria's physicians and medical professorate.

I remember one particular professor at the Pediatric University Hospital, where I completed my training. Communist Soviet-trained, he had a cold-eyed understanding of the problems facing his young patients. Rather than ask the hospital to replenish its supplies, he asked the clinical trainees under him to go out to the local pharmacies and buy up medications that were needful but had run out. Instead of an ethically and efficiently run pediatric unit, my Soviet-trained supervisor turned his hospital ward into a pharmaceutical black market, where prescriptions were sold privately, "under the table" to patients' families.

Indeed, "palms [had] to be greased for just about everything." If you were a family member of a patient, you couldn't just bring in food for your child. A guard would stop you at the front door. So you'd have to give him *baksheesh*—a "tip," in effect a bribe. A professor would tell parents that, in order for their children to be treated in hospital, they would first have to bring them to his private clinic for a consultation. The people visiting public hospitals were poor to begin with. If they had money, they would have gone in the first place to a private hospital where the care was usually (though not always) better. But while it was often better, it was also much more expensive, so only the well-to-do could afford private health care.

It's hard to imagine that professors would use their academic appointments to line their own pockets, but I suppose they weren't satisfied with the salaries paid in a socialist regime. So they spent their days trying to make money instead of making people well. They'd send patients to their own private clinics for unwarranted extra tests. They'd get kickbacks for prescribing MRIs and other expensive technologies. They'd get kickbacks from the hospital labs and even from surgeons and specialists to whom they referred patients.

Such was the state of medicine and of medical training in Assad's Syria. What follows next might seem a digression, but it's vital to my growth as a physician, teacher, and humanitarian.

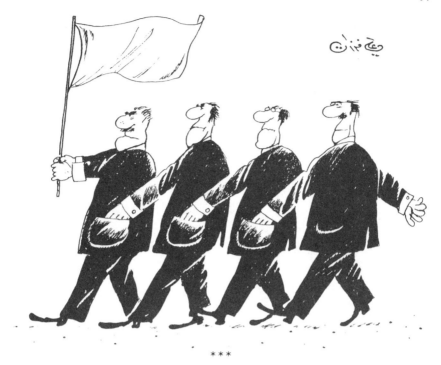

***

Throughout this memoir, I've focused on those moments when my world-view—as a young Sunni Arab growing up in Ba'athist Syria—was rattled and shocked and even cracked in some places (though not yet shattered). My first trip to the States, though lasting all of three weeks, was one of those moments. Sometimes, in order to see the world where you grew up and were taught the lessons of youth, you have to leave it. In leaving the Middle East for the first time as a young man, my eyes opened to a new world whose ways had no resemblance to Assad's Syria.

It was in the late summer of 1985. My father was going to visit his brother, my Uncle Bashar, who was Head of the Periodontology Department at the University of Minnesota Medical School in Minneapolis. I had saved enough money to cover expenses and my mother paid for my ticket, so I was going to tag along. More than my first trip outside of the Middle East, it would be my first visit to an American university, to an American hospital—to America. And what I experienced, from the moment that I got off the plane in Minneapolis, left me speechless.

It was August when my Dad and I arrived, and it was raining. I was enthralled. Here it was, summertime, and raining. That doesn't happen in summertime in Damascus. Even more magical than thunderstorms in summer

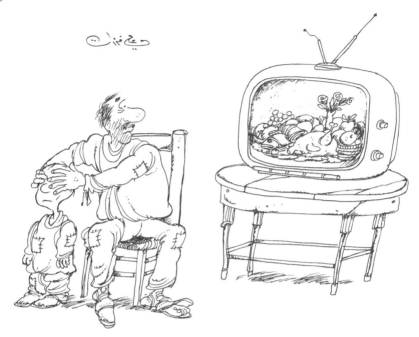

was the bounty brought by rain. The parks and lawns and lush greenery stretched out before me, as far as I could see. And so much fresh water! "The Land of 10,000 Lakes" is the nickname of Minnesota, and 10,000 lakes are about 9,999 more than we had in Damascus.

And with the summer rains came sweet corn, tomatoes larger than my clenched fists held together, zucchinis and squashes, and so many different melons, apples, pears. There were exotic fruits: bananas, mangoes, avocados. I love to eat and I've always enjoyed browsing in the bustling, fragrant outdoor markets of Damascus. In Minnesota, the markets were mostly indoors. They lacked some of the smells and some of the spices and produce I'd grown up eating. But what they did hold, all clean and neatly arranged, was a cornucopia of foods I had never before seen or imagined. It was in Minnesota that I learned what an American supermarket was like.

The first time I walked into Cup Foods Supermarket, my jaw dropped at the sight. Walls and aisles after aisles of the freshest produce, fresh and cured meats, dairy—so much dairy!—breads and sweets, and packaged goods. Each section or aisle was a world in itself. I remember walking slowly past the refrigerated display cases of seafood: fresh shrimp of all sizes, the oysters on ice, the colorful varieties of salmon and tuna (which I had never seen before), the tank of live lobsters. Remembering my Jordanian grandmother's feasts, the child in me delighted in the opulence and variety. The adult in me studied the contents of display cases in awesome silence, as if visiting a science lab or museum of technology.

When I visited my first indoor shopping mall I felt as if I had been dropped from outer space. Surely the superior technology of some alien race lay behind this "mothership" of stores, whose multi-leveled mall-tentacles reached out across acres of asphalt parking.

Please understand that I enjoy the sights and sounds and smells of Syria's outdoor markets. As I write this paragraph, I'm filled with nostalgia for Sha'alan, the neighborhood that lay between my home in the Malki district and my two-room private clinic in Damascus. Each work day I would walk past its produce stalls and food vendors, always stopping for a quick bite. But on this first trip to the States, standing in the epicenter of the Mall, I could not fight off the sense that this was the "modern world" that Ba'athist Syria had deliberately banished and hidden from its people. There where I stood, everything was new. Everything was fresh. Everything was orderly. Everything was clean.

There were no street-urchin beggars in the mall as in Sha'alan. The kids in the mall were washed, their hair neatly cut and combed. They wore shoes. They ran about but not too boisterously and answered when their mothers called. There were security guards, but they were polite and well-dressed and didn't carry AK-47s. There was no jostling. People smiled if you made eye contact. There were no scooters or fruit carts or cars to dodge. Above all, there was no dust kicked up from the dry Damascene summer. Back in Damascus, the daytime temperature hovered around 100° Fahrenheit. There in the air-conditioned mall, the temperature was a constant, cool seventy degrees.

Amazingly, no one seemed to notice or care that I was a Muslim. No one stopped and stared at me. If any family in that mall at that time were transported to Sha'alan, I can assure you that people would have stared. The beggars would have swooped down upon them and the vendors would have vied for their attention (and dollars), maybe even leading them by hand to their kiosks. Likely, a soldier or security agent would have followed their movements. But there, standing in the middle of the mall, I felt a glorious anonymity. No one cared who I was or what I was doing or why I was there—and that was fine by me.

The sensation that I wasn't being watched was likely an illusion. As I think about it, there must have been security cameras throughout the mall. But they weren't looking for me in particular, and I had no reason to fear them. I had absolutely no reason to fear the security guards, either. I was capable, perhaps for the first time in my life, of feeling that security guards were there to protect me, that I was safe in their midst, and that it's possible to live life without a pervasive sense of paranoia. That, in itself, was a revelation.

The rain, the greenery, the supermarkets, the shopping malls. All this, and my greatest shock was yet to come. Back in August, 1985, I was barely half-way through my medical studies in Damascus. When Uncle Bashar took me to visit the University of Minnesota Medical School, I was blown away—and not just by the facilities. What impressed me was the level of professionalism in all aspects of the teaching and practice of medicine.

After Uncle Bashar had given me an all-too-brief tour of the Medical School, it was my aunt Diane's turn to serve as chauffeur and tour guide. American born, aunt Diane worked as a nurse in a hospital affiliated with the Medical School. Once again, I was impressed by the facilities but more so by the staff. During my visit, her hospital was hosting a medical lecture, which she invited me to attend. Over the years, I've forgotten the lecture theme. What I haven't forgotten was the sense of professionalism that pervaded the affair. Everyone seemed so attentive and respectful to each other, I could hardly grasp that this was really happening. And aunt Diane gave me more than her time and attention. Knowing my need for books, she gave me a pharmaceutical handbook for nurses, which was a gold mine of information. I gathered up other books as well, to bring back with me. (As it turns out, I needed them to pass the US medical exams I'd one day take.)

Faculty at the University of Minnesota Medical School showed complete dedication to their students, whom they held to the highest standards and to whom they imparted the latest and best medical practice. There was no cronyism, no political favors, no Ba'athist parachuters in the University of Minnesota Medical School. Uncle Bashar held the positions he did because of merit—because of his training, experience, hard work, and devotion to his calling. This was a refreshing and hopeful insight. In mid-flight over the Atlantic Ocean, I resolved to further my studies and practice medicine in the US, regardless of obstacles I had to overcome to make that happen.

If I were to describe my final years in med school, I'd merely rehash the tawdry details already given. Suffice it to say that I finished the coursework and clinical training and was anxious to move on.

In America, graduating medical students take the Hippocratic Oath seriously. And, having since studied and practiced medicine in America, I've come to understand and appreciate the Oath's sacred character. But, back in Syria, the Oath of the Physician was just so many words you'd mouth before taking your diploma and starting your job. Back at the Damascus University

Medical School, they herded us into a room twenty at a time, had us raise our right hands, had us repeat the words, handed us our papers, and sent us off—quickly, for the next twenty in line. Sadly, this hurried, thoughtless, assembly-line approach to medical training was a perfect initiation into the Syrian health care system.

* * *

In a future chapter, I'll write of my experiences in America after medical school. Here, I should point out that I returned to Syria in 2002, both to teach in the Damascus University Medical School and to open up my own private clinic in pediatric neurology. Since I've focused much of this present chapter on the culture of graft present within the Syrian health system, I'd like to finish this theme before moving on.

It's not that I had forgotten al-Mousawat and its lessons in Ba'athist cronyism and corruption. What brought me back was "The Hope" (Lesch 2), as Syrians had taken to calling Hafez's second son, Bashar al-Assad. His presidency offered real prospects for a reformed, progressive Syria—and, Quixotically, I bought into that hope. So I returned to Damascus and opened my own little clinic, eager to contribute to this new, progressive Syria. But I soon learned that, when it came to Ba'athism, old habits die hard.

I remember my secretary entering my clinic office one afternoon. "A man wants to give you something, doctor," she said.

"Sure," I replied: "let him in."

The man entered, bowed slightly, and handed me an envelope. "What's in it?" I asked.

"Money, doctor," was his simple reply.

"For what?" was my simple reply.

"For your help in having your clinic order an MRI."

"That's taking a bribe," I said, affronted.

"Every physician does it," he answered. And I found that I couldn't fault him entirely, since he had been taught that health was purchased by *baksheesh*—the sort of bribe-taking that I had witnessed throughout my clinical training at al-Mouwasat.

The man had assumed that every physician took bribes, but I knew that this was not true. I did know several highly ethical, highly dedicated Syrian physicians who would give free consultations and would do surgeries for free if a patient couldn't afford it. In Damascus, there was a nonprofit organization called Sandook Al-Afia, meaning "Box of Hope." The donation boxes were simple affairs, made of cardboard with a piece of cloth placed inside. With little fanfare they were placed throughout the city, though mainly in the mosque complexes. And people knew what to do with them.

It was gratifying and humbling to see common Damascenes filling these boxes and giving so much for the welfare of others. I sent many of my own poorer patients to get help from the Sandook Al-Afia. Much of this charity came from people who had themselves suffered through the graft and indifference of the public health care system. God remembers and rewards acts of charity—which makes me wonder how my old med school professors (and others in Syria's broken health care system) will excuse their graft when God calls them to a final reckoning.

In my private practice from 2002 through 2010, I saw many Syrian children with neurological disorders. Their parents were rich and poor and in-between, but most were poor. And I was lucky to have donors ready to help. I, too, kept a box in my clinic, and it was never empty. The parents who brought their children in needed the help—and not just to pay for treatment. Some came from distant villages, traveling for as much as twelve hours, during which time they couldn't even change their children's diapers. You can imagine the smell. And many of these parents couldn't afford to buy diapers. Sometimes they'd improvise by spreading a piece of cloth inside a plastic shopping bag. And while some could afford the bus ride from their village to Damascus, often they didn't have the money to return.

And sometimes it wasn't financial help that was most needed. Sometimes it was simple human kindness—the prospect that someone in the Syrian medical community might actually *care* for the welfare of child and family.

I remember one day when five members of a family—two parents with their sick child, accompanied by two older men (a grandfather and uncle, I presume) came to my clinic from Deir ez-Zor, a province in the northeast of Syria currently controlled by ISIS. The mother placed in my hands an infant that had hydrocephalus—a dangerous buildup of excess fluid in the head. At the same time, the grandfather placed a small stack of Syrian pounds on my examining table. I recorded the child's medical history and proceeded to examine her.

"I am sorry," I said to the mother, handing back her infant. Of course the adults gathered in my small examining room listened intently, too. "Your child has hydrocephalus, which I am not equipped to treat. You will need to visit a specialist. Here," I said, writing down contact information for a specialist in hydrocephaly. "I recommend that you see Dr Joukhadar. He's a fine neurosurgeon and a good man and he will do his best to treat your child."

"And here," I continued, picking up the money that had been placed on my examination table. It amounted to 500 Syrian pounds (the equivalent, at the time, of ten US dollars). "Take this back. And may your child be cured, *inshallah*."

The family left. Several minutes later, one of the men came back—the uncle, as I imagined him. "Please, let me shake your hand," he asked of me, extending his own hand.

"Sure," I said, trying to hide my confusion. As we shook hands, he continued speaking.

"I am a district judge," he said, "and I never thought I would see such an act by a doctor in Syria. You gave us our money back, which was the right thing to do."

"You make me happy," I replied, "but also sad, if doing the right thing has become so rare as you say."

I remember another case, a child that had a progressive and incurable neurological disease. A few months after I had last treated the child, a man came into my office unannounced and without an appointment. It was the father of the child. "My daughter has died," he said, and my immediate thought was that he was going to vent his anger on me. But he didn't.

"Here," he said, handing me a package.

"What is it?" I asked, still a bit unnerved.

"It's a gift, doctor," he said. "I want to thank you for being there for my family when we needed you and for telling us the truth about our daughter's condition." It was a small token accompanying a letter that elaborated on his expression of thanks.

I still have that letter. This was *baksheesh* as God intended it to be practiced. As a token of gratitude, not as a bribe. The man had nothing to gain by visiting me. He had already suffered the loss of his child. But he took time to come back and say thanks. His action humbled me, and it also reminded me that kindness breeds kindness, even in Assad's Syria.

And yet, individual acts of kindness achieve little when an entire nation despairs. Take everything that I've been describing—the widespread poverty and lack of resources, the institutionalized cronyism and incompetence, the pervasive culture of graft—and add decades of regional warfare.

In 2003, American President George W. Bush invaded Iraq in search of "weapons of mass destruction." He did not find them. Apparently, they did

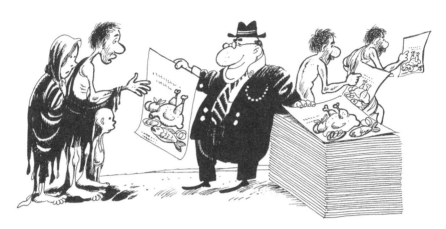

not exist. But there was, indeed, "mass destruction" in Syria's Ba'athist neighbor, and some 2,000,000 Iraqis sought refuge in my country. In my private clinic, I treated many Iraqi children who were among these war refugees. I remember one sweet seven-year-old girl, whose mother had brought her to my clinic. When I next saw the child, she was brought in by her uncle. Curious, I asked about her mother. "She was killed by a bomb," the uncle replied. I looked down at the child's face, speechless.

Sometimes it was the children who spoke, and the stories they told were so sad. Some had lost a father or mother or both parents together. A stray bullet, a piece of shrapnel, a shattering window pane. The very randomness of their parents' deaths was heart-sickening. I felt helpless, since the wounds these children suffered were psychological as much as physical. Even back then I asked myself, *"How will they grow up, having witnessed so much violence? How will war scar them?"*

And now, some eleven years later, these war-traumatized children have grown into young men and women. Who among them will have forgotten, much less forgiven, the forces that destroyed their homes and families? And who among them will be fighting right now, on one or other side of Iraq's Sunni-ISIS-Shia conflict?

I admit that this chapter has jumped back and forth across many dates, from 1983 to 1985, 1988, 2002, 2010, and 2014. But much of the foundation for today's Syrian/Iraqi crisis was laid in those years. While I've been writing about the failed Syrian health care system, it should be obvious that I'm describing an endemic *political* failure. While the rise of ISIS has complicated matters severely, I remain convinced that Ba'athism is the major disease afflicting Syria, its hospitals, and its schools today. And, even should the civil war end tomorrow, the nation's health care woes will only have gotten worse since 2010, when I left for the States for good.

Clearly, the Syrian people's collective health won't improve until the nation's politics improves. It's always the poorest that are the most oppressed and have most to gain from regime change. And this fact should help American readers understand the rise of sectarian political parties throughout the Arab world. Remember the Sandook Al-Afia or "Box of Hope." The region's mosques, and not its government agencies, have been the major source of help for the poor. Taking the next logical step, I would say that religious fundamentalism is a consequence of the failure of secular (and, in the Ba'athist case, of Soviet-style fascist) government to provide basic human services. The only "lawful" secular authority in Assad's Syria, the Ba'ath Party, has proved itself the people's enemy, not their protector. So it's not surprising that people give their loyalty to the Imams.

The mosques and their Imams have been and continue to be a force for good in Syria, despite the actions and attitudes of a radicalized minority who justify violence through distorted readings of the Quran. What concerns me deeply is that ISIS has taken over the traditional, charitable role of the mosque in some Sunni villages. If you're hungry and an Islamist hands you bread, you'll take it and thank him. The bread will have bought your loyalty. Soon your village will be under ISIS control. And then the Islamic State's brand of brutal, medieval "justice" will sweep through your village, cleansing it of "heretics" and "infidels" (your one-time neighbors, with whom you had lived and worked in peace). And anything that smacks of "Western" secularism and decadence will be smashed. Such is the power of bread to buy the hungry man's allegiance, his passive assent, and ultimately his loss of freedom.

5
Leaving Syria Forever
(For the First Time)

> Whoso emigrates in the way of God will find in the earth many
> refuges and plenty.
>
> —Quran 4: 100).

When I finished Damascus University Medical School in September, 1988,
I felt as if I had finished a six-year prison sentence. The day after gradua-
tion, I began the paperwork to leave for the United States. The so-called
Supervision Department of the Ba'ath Party didn't make it easy for non-party
members to apply for study or medical residency abroad. Keep in mind that
Syria had compulsory military service, so a graduate of Damascus University
Medical School either continued his studies or put on an army uniform.
Members of the Ba'ath Party had an easier time of it. As a reward for loyalty,
the party would send graduates off to an Eastern Bloc country where they'd
learn the language and continue their medical studies tuition-free. Some
went to Romania or Bulgaria, but most went to the Soviet Union where they
learned to speak Russian and practice medicine.

Some Ba'athist graduates whose families could afford it studied in France
or the UK. Bashar al-Assad belonged to the latter group. In 1992, President
Hafez al-Assad's second son entered London's Western Eye Hospital as a post-
graduate student in ophthalmology. Obviously, Hafez could afford the out-
of-state tuition. Keep in mind that Hafez's oldest son and "heir apparent,"
Bassel, was alive at the time. Bashar—or, rather, Colonel Bashar al-Assad, for
he had begun his medical residency at the Tishreen Military Hospital—remained in London until his brother's death in 1994, when he was called back
to military service in Syria.

Again, the Supervision Department usually approved a party member's application to study in the West, so long as he or she could afford it. But most
graduates of Damascus University couldn't afford it. Besides, most of them
couldn't dream of passing a real exam given in a real medical school in France
or the UK. (You'll remember that a majority of my fellow graduates got into

medical school through party loyalty and not through native wit.) For these loyal Ba'athists, the Syrian government offered an expenses-paid indoctrination in Soviet-style health care.

This should explain why I've implicated the Soviet Union in Syria's failed health care system. Having completed their studies and residency in a Communist nation whose health care has been ranked 130th by the World Health Organization, they returned to practice and teach medicine in a nation whose health care was ranked 108th. These Soviet-trained physicians filled the Ba'athist Syrian professorate, ensuring a uniform mediocrity up and down the ranks of academia. And, as a further indoctrination in Soviet-style leadership, they returned with an expertise in graft that placed economic self-interest ahead of the education of students and the welfare of patients.

For those of us who weren't loyal Ba'athists, study abroad meant a mountain of paperwork. That, in itself, was hardly surprising, since government review and approval was required for virtually every transaction of any consequence. What made the process so anxious for my non-Ba'athist fellows was how steeply the odds were stacked against them. In most dealings with the government, one knows that decisions will be arbitrary and capricious, reflecting the sheer indifference of the people behind the desk: "The answer's 'no,' but it's nothing personal," is something that a Syrian gets used to hearing. But, when it came to dealings with the Supervision Department, the

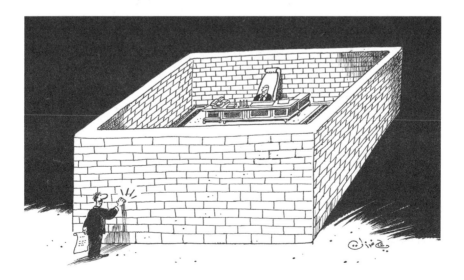

answer was "no" more often than "yes," and any applicant for study in the West—especially in the States—would fall under serious scrutiny.

So, most of my friends and fellow graduates could only dream of leaving Syria for the West. What made me an incredibly lucky exception was that I already had my green card—which meant that I didn't have to run the deadly gauntlet of a visa application. I received it in 1985, when I was twenty. You'll remember that my father and I had visited my uncle Bashar, who taught and practiced at the University of Minnesota Medical School in Minneapolis. Because of that trip, I had my card—my magic carpet to fly out of Syria, once and for all.

Still, the number of stamps and signatures needed from so many different governmental offices was mind-boggling. With each added stamp and signature, my excitement grew in anticipation of leaving. But with each passing day, the fear grew, too. What if the Supervision Department denied my application? All it would take would be for one person to say I had done something or said something against the government—something as harmless as a joke poking fun at Hafez could keep me in Damascus or, worse, land me in the Syrian Army Medical Corps. It felt schizophrenic, this bouncing between excitement and fear. The fear was paranoid, I admit. But, in Assad's Syria, paranoia was a part of daily life. If you think someone's watching, someone probably is.

Until the Supervision Department approved your application, you'd be treated like a suspect in a crime. But, once your application was approved, you'd be treated like Ba'athist family. They'd let you buy as many as 500 US dollars at a special rate of four Syrian pounds per dollar. Back in 1988, greenbacks sold on the black market for eleven pounds per dollar. Of course, they were trying their best to ingratiate themselves with the physicians going abroad. I assume they were afraid we'd never come back. If so, their fears were well founded. I'd guess that nine in ten physicians who left Syria for the States never returned. Why would they want to?

So, I had my green card in hand and my papers in order, all signed and stamped. I was ready to pack my bags—as good as gone. And then came the official announcement. The Syrian government would not be allowing any graduates to leave the country. I panicked. I went to my parents and told them I had to leave, the very next day if possible, for Jordan where my cousins lived. My chances of studying in the US hung by a thread. No Syrian physician could leave without the government's formal, official approval.

The night before I left, I told two close friends and no one else. When I

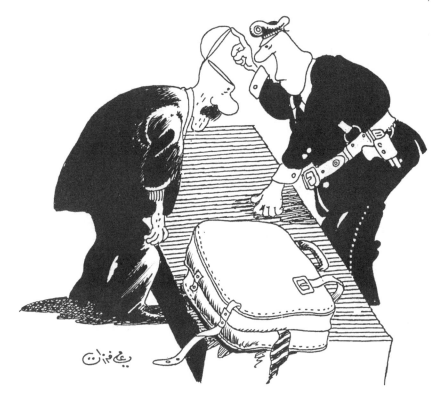

went to the Damascus airport to fly to Jordan, I felt like a spy on the run—someone whose cover had been blown. I thought that I knew what paranoia felt like. Nothing I had experienced heretofore approached the dread that I felt while standing in line at the ticket counter. I wasn't just leaving, I was escaping.

Ticket in hand, I headed to the first security check point. Beyond that point, only passengers could pass. So my mother, who had come with me, could go no farther. We hugged and kissed, but she was not ready to let go. Reaching up, she pulled my head down to hers and held on, planting kisses while giving the usual motherly admonitions and instructions, crying all the while. But my flight time was approaching and I said my final, heartfelt good-bye and blessing. I turned to the agent who checked my ticket and passed into the "security zone" of the airport.

I was walking in a daze, so intent on my own thoughts that I did not hear the second security guard ask for my passport. "Are you deaf?" the agent yelled: "the sergeant wants to see your passport!" I have heard of people being so scared that they'd soil themselves. I didn't, but I felt that moment as if I could. Thank goodness the sergeant was kinder: "Let him be," he said: "Can't you see he just said goodbye to his crying mother?" Of course, it was more than my mother that I was saying goodbye to.

I boarded the plane, took my seat, and buckled in. When the plane began to lift off the runway and the force of gravity shoved me back against my seat, I didn't feel my usual gut-feeling of fear on take-off. For once, I was ex-ultant. "They can't stop me now!" I thought. Looking out the cabin window at Damascus, I remember saying to myself, "I swear never to return to Syria." What a solemn, sad vow for a young man to make over his native land.

When the plane landed in Amman, Jordan, I declared myself a free man. I had snapped the chains binding me to Assad's Syria. What I hadn't counted on was the level of airport security on the other side of the border.

As passengers walked single file through the terminal gate, I was asked to step out of line and join the group of Syrians who had just deplaned. There were a number of us, since it was a flight from Damascus. Still, the request seemed ominous. My first thought, of course paranoid, was that the *mukhabarat*—the Syrian Military Intelligence Directorate—had found me out. The Syrian Military Intelligence Directorate had asked its Jordanian counterparts to seize me and send me back to face punishment—horrid pun-ishment, no doubt—for going AWOL. In a matter of minutes, I had gone from a freed man to a military prisoner. My second thought was almost as paranoid. Relations between Syria's President Assad and Jordan's King Hussein had gone sour of late. Maybe Jordanian security suspected us of being spies, militants, or traffickers. Or maybe the Jordanian government was simply venting its anger on its northern neighbor by hassling its citizens. Whatever their reason, members of the Jordanian airport security started in on their interrogations.

They began with an old merchant from Aleppo. "I flew through Amman just last week!" he declared, incredulous: "I've flown through Amman hun-dreds of times! I am a simple, honest merchant. Traveling is my livelihood. I've traveled as a merchant for forty years!" The Jordanian security weren't impressed by his pleas and they kept him in custody, moving him over to what seemed like a holding area for customs violators and illegal immigrants.

Soon it was my turn, and I found myself standing before the chief inter-rogator for airport security. He was a thin man about my height, dressed formally in a tie. He didn't wear the khaki uniform and beret of the Royal Jordanian army. He was definitely Jordanian, not Palestinian: Palestinians weren't allowed to hold such official, powerful jobs. His questions came in rapid-fire succession—I had barely begun answering one before he was on to the next.

"What are you doing in Jordan?"

"What political party do you belong to?"

"Where are you staying in Amman?"

Though he pressed on aggressively, I was eager to answer that last question: "I'll be spending time with my family before continuing on the United States" so, while I had a tiny opening, I blurted out, "with the Khaleefeh family."

"So, your family is Jordanian?" he boomed out, his words more like a declaration than a question. It's as if he were pronouncing magic words that opened an otherwise locked door.

"Yes, Jordanian," I replied, trying to sound and appear calm though I was visibly shaking: "I have family all over Amman."

At once he was all smiles, clapping me on the back in welcome. "Why didn't you say so from the beginning!" he said, jocularly. He gave me a friendly push on my way, as if pleased to find a fellow countryman among this rabble of suspicious Syrians. And I made good time in separating myself from the rest of his abject detainees. I glanced back at the bewildered old merchant from Aleppo, who sat nervously in custody. He was glaring at me, jealously and indignantly.

* * *

I always enjoyed my visits to relatives in Amman, but this visit was especially sweet. When I first arrived, I stayed with cousin Samaar, her husband, and their eighteen-month-old son, Omar. Every morning, Omar would come over to the mattress I was sleeping on over in my corner of the living room floor. Summoned from the depths of sleep, I'd feel a warm, moist, milk-laden breath on my face. That became my early-morning alarm clock. Omar was a very cute child, though I should note that he's grown now and become an engineer. Every morning, Omar would beg for "mar," expecting me to get a small container of the Turkish strawberry jam that his Dad sold and feed it to him with a spoon. It wasn't the most nutritious breakfast, but it was certainly tasty. When I felt that hot, milky breath on my face and heard the child's voice crooning "Mar, mar, mar" (the first syllable of "marmalade"), I knew my slumber was finished and my day begun.

My plan was to study for ECFMG Certification. The Philadelphia-based

Educational Commission for Foreign Medical Graduates serves as a national clearinghouse for schools and foreign medical students. I've just surfed the ECFMG website and found its mission statement:

> The ECFMG promotes quality health care for the public by certifying international medical graduates for entry into US graduate medical education, and by participating in the evaluation and certification of other physicians and health care professivonals nationally and internationally.[14]

The website gives an interesting stat. One in four physicians currently practicing in the States attended foreign medical school—so I'm not alone by any stretch of the imagination. Physicians the world over want to come to the States to pursue their advanced studies. And, once they've proved themselves, they want to stay.

And that was my goal. To get more fluent in English, get ECFMG certified, get to the States, get a medical residency, and get a job—a logical progression. The University of Jordan was in walking distance from my cousin's apartment, so I planned to settle into its library and start studying.

But now, freed from every constraint—and every incentive—that family, school, and community had placed on me, I experienced something I had never allowed myself to feel before. Yes, I did go to the University library to study, and I did study, somewhat. But, for once in my adult life, I felt free to rest and relax and even enjoy myself a bit. And, the closer I came to know my other cousin Reem and her Jordanian and Palestinian friends, the easier it became to lay my books aside and luxuriate over conversation and coffee—especially when cousin Sahar's female friends came over.

At home in Damascus and at Al-Thaqafi School, my life was structured around my studies. Not only my parents, but my brother and friends had come to expect this of me. I was supposed to be the top student in my class, and I was not going to disappoint. Damascus University was far less challenging than Al-Thaqafi, so I had less need to apply myself. I wasn't aware of it, but my study habits had already begun to slip.

One morning, as I was walking to the library, I heard people chanting for Yasser Arafat. It was 1988, and the PLO leader had been in exile in Tunis since 1982. I assume they were Palestinian students attending the University of Jordan. "We will sacrifice our souls and blood for you, Arafat!" they cried out repeatedly.

Then I heard a counterpoint to their chanting. A bit farther down the street, a group of young Jordanians—students, I assume, at the University—were chanting with an equal fervor, "We will sacrifice our souls and blood for you, King Hussein!"

"*Great!*" I thought to myself: "*free speech, a campus march—this is what democracy is all about!*" I had never witnessed a demonstration before, with two factions squaring off in public. But the spectacle soon turned bloody. The Jordanians had brought sticks along with their slogans. Racing up to their fellow students, they began beating them mercilessly. The Palestinians didn't fight back. Their only weapons had been words, and when the Jordanian students attacked, the Palestinian students covered their heads with their hands and scattered. Seeking cover, they ran into campus buildings and shut the doors. It could have ended there, but the Jordanian students ran after them. If a door was locked or barricaded, they broke it down, pulled the Palestinians out of hiding, and beat them again.

There were Jordanian police everywhere, but they stood by, watching. I suppose they were watching to make sure the Palestinians didn't fight back. None of the Palestinians fought. Had one of them thrown a punch, I suspect that the police would have "come to the rescue" of their Jordanian fellow citizen and administered their own, more professional brand of beating.

I left the scene, horrified. The Palestinian students had been loud but peaceful in their demonstration. I didn't like Yasser Arafat myself, but so what? Let the students chant their PLO slogans. So long as they didn't block traffic or disturb people's sleep, how were they harming anyone? I left Syria to find freedom, and it saddened me to think that Jordan was no better.

I understand that these were radicalized factions squaring off. Not every Palestinian offered his blood for Arafat, not every Jordanian offered her blood for Hussein—my cousin Reem's circle of friends taught me that. Religion and politics laid aside, nothing kept Jordanians and Palestinians and Syrians from lounging together over conversation and a cup of Arabic coffee.

What saddens me now, as I think back to this event, is that I, too, stood passively by, watching. I don't know what I could have done, other than throw myself on top of one of the Palestinians in some gesture of protection. Likely, I would have been beaten in his place. Even if I chose not to act in that way, what troubles me is that I never thought to act at all. Throughout my life in Syria, I was taught to look away when someone in power abused that power. If someone carried a weapon I was taught to look down. Every time I walked past the rich houses in the rich neighborhood beyond my apartment building, I kept my eyes squarely on the ground before me, never looking up. It's a weird variation of "What you don't know can't hurt you. What you don't see won't hurt you."

The events of that day might have steeled my resolve to leave for the States, but, in fact, I stayed in Amman from October, 1988 to early March, 1989. Not wanting to wear out my welcome at cousin Samaar's, I moved from one cousin's home to another. They were each so generous and kind that I remain in their debt, even to this day. They certainly weren't judgmental about this newly-trained physician who, instead of practicing medicine, spent his days studying and flirting—or was it flirting and studying?—with coeds at the University of Jordan.

Having taken the first ECFMG exam, the time had at last come for me to fly to the States. My cousin Nuha, a Palestinian widow with three young girls to take care of, kindly welcomed me into her Michigan home. In a gesture that somehow signaled my severance from Syria and the Middle East, I shaved my beard, keeping only my mustache. When I phoned my mother and told her, she began crying. She loved my beard and had never seen my adult face without it. And now I was beardless, somehow different from the Syrian son she had raised.

And, soon, I had a second phone call to make it even more tearful for my mother. I had gotten my test results back from the ECFMG exam. I failed it. Not by much, but I failed it nonetheless. And I had only myself to blame. Back in Amman, had I spent more time studying and less time flirting with coeds, I would have passed it with ease.

My mother was devastated by my failure, and so was I. So I got out my books and vowed that this next time, thoroughly prepared, I would ace the exam. Still, the stark reality of my situation hit home with greater fury. Here I was, facing the end of winter in Michigan. For all the time I had spent visiting the American School in Damascus, I could not conceal the fact that I was a stranger in a strange land. And, having failed the ECFMG exam, I was facing a scary, unknown future.

Once I got over the shocks of failure and foreignness and settled into my studies, I began to feel "at home." An old friend of my brother's, Nouri, was living in Detroit, and we decided to become roommates. The street we lived on was close to Eight Mile Road, which separated the predominately African-American inner city from suburban white communities north of Detroit. The community that we lived in was—to my great comfort and delight—filled with Syrians. In most American states, Spanish is the most common second language. But in Michigan, it's Arabic. I felt like I was living in a wintery version of Damascus, with all the traditional Syrian talk, food, and clothing—and even an occasional hookah.

Though the culture of our community was Syrian, still there were differences between Detroit and Damascus. Detroit, after all, was the automobile capital of the world. And, unlike Damascus, you needed a car to get around. My first automotive venture was an old Buick Skylark, which I bought for $600. Yes, it was a cheap price and, yes, I got what I paid for. It broke down almost immediately and, instead of driving it, my friends and I wound up pushing it to a service station where it cost another $300 to get it repaired. There was a hole in the floor of the driver's side, which I covered with a piece of carpet. It drove for about six months, and then one day it just stopped. I supposed it had died of old age.

I had already started my medical residency at the Henry Ford Hospital. Since I had no earthly idea how cars worked, I asked a fellow resident to check out my cheap, old, dead Buick. She was kind enough to take a look at the engine. She popped the hood and let out a terrified scream. We found out why my car had died. A big, fat Detroit rat had moved in. Apparently it was fond of rubber-coated wiring, because it chewed the engine wires beyond the point of repair.

Automotively, God was kind to me when another Syrian, also looking for a better life in the US, called to offer me a deal. He had a much older car, a 1978 Chrysler Imperial, which he was selling for the amazingly low price of 175 bucks. I tried in a spirited way to haggle the price down but failed. It was a titanic silver monster that actually drove very smoothly. And I felt so safe inside it! I never opened the hood for the entire year I had it, until I sold it to another Syrian for the same price. For once, automotive karma was working in my favor.

I've already noted that I was interning at Henry Ford Hospital, so it's obvious that I had passed the ECFMG Certification exam on my second go-round. But that's not to say that the second time was easier or less stressful than the first. Within our Syrian community, several other recent med school graduates had arrived, each with the intention of taking the ECFMG. Since none of us really had a clue how to study for the exam, we enrolled in the Kaplan Center in Detroit. We went to the Center every weekday. It was an anxious time of my life, not knowing if I'd succeed. But, being there with other Syrian doctors who were equally anxious of the future gave some consolation.

Though we were students together at Kaplan, I can't say that we were boon companions. Our little community was a composite of Syrian society back home—meaning that our ethnic and religious prejudices had accompanied us to the States. Back in the Middle East, the Lebanese Civil War was raging. Here in Detroit, a Lebanese Maronite Christian spoke vehemently in support of the Israeli occupation of the south. His vehemence was matched by the Sunni Muslims, both Lebanese and Syrian, who supported the PLO. And then the Sunnis had their occasional words with a Shiite. So, here we were, arguing over religion and politics—just like back home. Unlike back home, we shared the Kaplan facilities with several Russian Jewish immigrants. Needless to say, *we* never spoke to *them*, and *they* never tried to speak to *us*.

Our prejudices, though rancorous, offered little more than an occasional distraction from the work at hand. We completed our studies and passed our exams and went our separate ways, though I didn't go far at all, having been accepted as a resident in Detroit's Henry Ford Hospital.

***

In February, 1990, just as I was preparing for residency at the hospital, Saddam Hussein sent his Iraqi legions steamrolling over its oil-rich but militarily feeble southern neighbor, Kuwait. My Palestinian cousins and Syrian friends weren't all that surprised. Hussein had already amassed what at that time was the world's fourth largest army on the Kuwaiti border. And he was making demands. Iraq's economy was in shambles from the Iran-Iraq War and Hussein's regime owed billions to the Kuwaiti royal family. While Iraq was impoverishing itself through war, the Al-Sabah family was busy multiplying its already enormous wealth.

The Kuwaiti royal family had ingratiated itself with the US government by replacing Iran as a supplier of cheap oil—and, by selling oil at a discount to Americans, the Kuwaitis were effectively deflating world oil prices. Iraq needed money to rebuild, and that money would have to come from oil sales. Iraq tried to bully Kuwait into forgiving its war debt and raising the price of crude. When Kuwait resisted, the Iraqi dictator took it personally, making it a "matter of honor" to punish the Kuwaitis for their insolence.

Didn't Saddam personally lead the Sunni cause against the Iranian Shia revolution? Weren't the Kuwaitis guilty of stealing Iraqi oil by "slant drilling" into its northern neighbor's oil fields? And wasn't the very formation of Kuwait an imposition of the British mandate—a mistake on the map of the Middle East? When Kuwait declared its independence in 1961, Iraq had reason to object, declaring this collection of tiny, oil-rich islands little more than an Iraqi province. And now, some thirty years later, Hussein was bent on "correcting" that political error and returning Kuwait to the Iraqi fold. These are not my arguments, needless to say. These were the rationalizations of an Iraqi dictator who saw Kuwaiti wealth as a solution to his nation's battered economy.

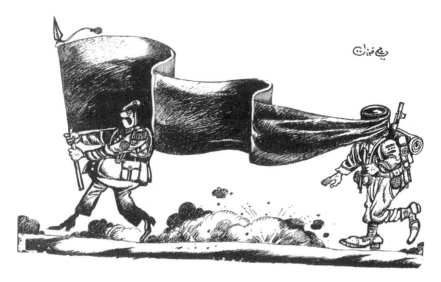

You might think that a wave of outrage passed through Detroit's Syrian community at Iraq's invasion of a sovereign, fellow-Sunni nation. But my Palestinian cousins and most of my Syrian friends took it as so much "business as usual." They were unpersuaded by the fact that eleven Arab states—including Egypt, Turkey, Pakistan, Saudi Arabia and, yes, Assad's Syria—had joined the US in a thirty-four nation coalition against Hussein. "After all," they'd say, "it was the flow of oil," and not the defense of freedom, that brought this coalition together. The US was protecting its economic interests. In liberating Kuwait, the coalition forces would be restoring a monarchy, not building democracy. And my cousins owed no allegiance to the Al-Sabah family. What had Kuwait done to help solve the Palestinian refugee crisis? I would have expected my cousins to show some sympathy toward a conquered people. Instead, playing the victim-game of "haves" vs "have nots," several seemed to take some grim satisfaction in seeing the rich Kuwaitis humbled: "So, now *they* know what foreign occupation feels like." It's not that my cousins took pleasure in the invasion and its inherent injustice. I think they were reacting out of the conviction that their lands had been taken and their rights trampled on, but no US-led coalition would ever come to their aid. In fact, they seemed to place some faint hope in Hussein's brash declaration of the forthcoming "Mother of All Battles" as if the Iraqi occupation of Kuwait could in any way help the Palestinian cause.

When Hussein declared his intention to shoot Scuds at Israel, that pretty much sealed the deal. "*Let this be the Mother of All Battles,*" my Palestinian cousins must have thought, "*nothing else has helped.*" (But it didn't help. Fired from their jobs and harassed by Iraqi occupation forces, Palestinians fled Kuwait in the tens of thousands. It's always the weakest who suffer the worst.)

My Syrian friends directed their heaviest cynicism at Hafez al-Assad. There was nothing noble in the behind-the-scenes bargaining that brought Syria into the war. A coalition-defeated Iraq would increase Syria's regional power and give Assad a freer hand in Lebanon. And Hafez had long suspected Saddam of making attempts on his life. So it was the usual mixture of ambition, paranoia, and self-interest that brought Syria into the coalition.

Of all the wars I had experienced up to this point in my life, this one had to have been the most senseless. It was bound to fail, and fail disastrously. Seduced by power, dictators may develop delusions of grandeur. But, surely, their survival instincts must also be pretty strong. (Even Hitler might have hung on had he settled for the *Sudetenland* rather than the whole of Eastern Europe.) The Iraqi invasion of Kuwait was sheer suicide. How could Hussein not have known that?

I remember watching TV shortly after the Iraqi conquest of Kuwait. Saddam Hussein was in Baghdad, filmed in what seemed to be a hotel lobby full of Western "guests," mostly European. They had the misfortune of being in Baghdad when the invasion occurred, and their presence was of considerable value—not as guests, but as hostages. The Iraqi cameras showed Saddam talking to a young British boy, asking him if he was getting his milk. I recall him addressing the boy by name—Stewart—in a solicitous way, like a kindly uncle.

Of course, there was a double message to this grotesque, staged interview. On the one hand, "little Stewart" was being kept safe and sound in a luxurious Baghdad hotel. Such was the generosity of Saddam Hussein to the citizens of countries that were even then lining up against him. On the other hand, "little Stewart" had become a military asset as valuable as a reinforced bunker. Like Saddam's other European "guests," he provided a "human shield" in the event of a Western attack. In the days before Operation Desert Storm (January 17, 1991—February 28, 1991), I have a memory of Saddam giving daily photo-ops with "human shields" occasionally in the background, as if part of his entourage.

Before Operation Desert Storm there was Operation Desert Shield (August 2, 1990—January 17, 1991), when the United States scurried to deploy deterrent forces in Saudi Arabia and throughout the Gulf region. Over these six months, it seemed like "all quiet on the Mid-Eastern Front." Then all hell broke loose. On January 17, a blistering aerial bombardment began that lasted for five weeks. "The Mother of All Battles" was at hand. I do not know what happened to "Little Stewart," though I trust that he wasn't part of the bombardment's "collateral damage." The coalition air forces had six months to plan their sorties, and their missiles and "smart bombs" largely missed the hotels where foreign "guests" and news reporters were staying.

When Desert Shield turned to Desert Storm, I was riveted to the TV set, as were virtually all of my Syrian friends—and many Americans, too. In the past, I had seen televised footage of battles and their aftermath. I had listened to radio reports and read newspapers. But never before had I seen war televised continuously live, as CNN was doing. I remember the CNN night-vision cameras filming the Baghdad skyline. From the ground, streams of antiaircraft cannon fire (largely ineffective) would start to crackle and a CNN reporter would hold his microphone out the hotel window to capture the sound. Soon, a missile would streak down from the sky, blasting into a building—to be followed by a bomb, and then another missile, and then another bomb.

Those early days and nights of news coverage were mesmerizing to watch: eerie, surreal—so fascinating that one almost forgot the human cost. During the Vietnam War, American TV coverage fueled anti-war sentiment. Likely, Hussein was hoping for much the same impact. But the images broadcast by CNN had an entirely different effect. There were no close-up camera shots of soldiers or civilians on the ground. The ground assault was still some weeks away. It was the technology, not the humanity, of war that was put on display. And it did not take long for the Iraqis to realize that the TV coverage showed only the awesome power and efficiency of the coalition forces as they flew 100,000 sorties in a mere few weeks, dropping countless thousands of tons of ordinance on Iraqi targets.

I remember the coalition commander, American General Norman Schwartzkopf, giving a televised briefing that included a "bomb's-eye view" of the bombardment. One video showed a "smart bomb" as it arced through the air with the televised cross-hairs on a rapidly approaching Iraqi tank that it blew to smithereens. Another video was taken from the cockpit of a jet. There was the ground target—a building of some strategic importance—the missile fired, and then the explosion as the missile slammed into the center, hitting the bull's eye.

It was bizarre to watch and read about Desert Storm. Despite the size and the quality of the forces arrayed against them, the Iraqis were a formidable army, well dug-in. They had six months to prepare for the defense of Kuwait, just as the coalition had six months to prepare for the assault. The Iraqis had held out for years against Iran. Who would have predicted that the

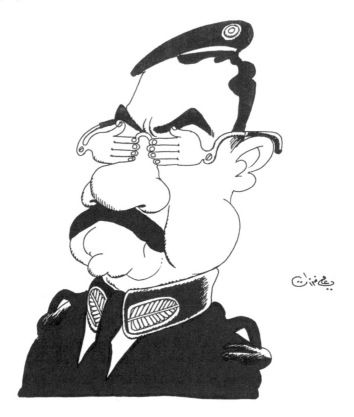

ground battle for Kuwait would last just one hundred hours? Probably the most compelling image of the entire war was the burned out hulks of tanks and armored transports that littered the "highway of death." In their haste to retreat from Kuwait, the Iraqi forces had created a sixty-kilometer long traffic jam along the desert road leading from Kuwait City back to Baghdad. The coalition jets annihilated the retreating tanks—it was like target practice.

It was during the TV coverage of Operation Desert Storm that I spoke, for the first time, of my change of heart toward war. I remember sitting with my Palestinian cousins, Suad and Eiad, and hearing the reports of Hussein's rocket-firing against Israel. The rockets were an attempt to goad Israel into a military response that would turn popular Arab sentiment against the coalition. The rockets managed to do some damage and some seventy Israelis were killed. My cousins were ecstatic whenever a missile hit Israeli territory, as if their favorite soccer team had scored a goal.

"Why are you cheering the deaths of civilians?" I asked my cousins. They looked at me in puzzlement.

"Tarif, he's hitting the *enemy*," they replied.

"No," I replied: "he's killing innocent civilians. You cannot reach justice through injustice. In our lifetime, war has never solved anything. War is the enemy. The only path to justice is through peace, not war."

My cousins looked as if they had been slapped in the face. "Tarif," cousin Eiad said, trying to speak calmly: "*Who are you?* I don't know you anymore."

Truth was, I barely knew myself at that moment. The Tarif that I was becoming was too new even for me to understand fully. This was the first time that I had said such things, and possibly the first time that I had thought these things with such clarity and decisiveness. I wasn't just speaking to my Palestinian cousins, I was listening to my own words, as if they were being spoken by a person to whom I had just been introduced. And I was determined to make this person's acquaintance and to become friends with him, this new Tarif, if possible.

What I didn't tell my cousins, since I was only then learning this new truth about myself, was that religious and ethnic hatred was losing its hold over me. Even before I began work at Henry Ford, the process of unlearning had begun that would loosen hatred's hold upon me. My work at Henry Ford sped up the process, and the Gulf War had given me my first occasion to speak it out loud to the world.

I have witnessed other wars and have written of my confusion and shame in the wake of Arab defeat. I was taught to feel that shame over the Six-Day War and I felt it directly in aftermath of the Yom Kippur War. In the past, I would have felt anger and embarrassment at the swift collapse of Hussein's army and its ignominious retreat down the "highway of death." But my response to this event had nothing to do with failed or misplaced patriotism. I lamented, not the defeat of an Arab army at the hands of a superior military technology, but the profound waste of human life. It was not as Arabs, but as fellow human beings that their deaths deserved mourning. If the Iraqi army had been built in the same Ba'athist manner as Syria's, then I can guarantee that many, perhaps most, of the soldiers who died did so through a compelled valor. They were not given a chance to surrender. They were not given a chance to say no. They were victims of an ideology that sent them off to do battle and left them to their deaths. I mourned their humanity. For the first time in my life, I saw a Middle East war as a human tragedy, and not as an Arab defeat. Transcending pan-Arab ideology and the Ba'athist teachings of my youth, I had, at last, become a humanitarian.

Let me state now how I arrived at this change of heart.

* * *

I've made it clear that my hatred for Israel, Israelis, and Jews in general was part of the Syrian Ba'athist school curriculum. They were the enemy. No Syrian would have any doubt or ambivalence about that fact. Our identities rested firmly upon the bedrock of that hatred. And we were sure that all Israelis felt the same about us. Jew and Muslim, Israeli and Arab, were like oil and water—or should I say oil and fire.

And, as I've noted, we exported our prejudices when immigrating to the States. But greater Detroit was not little Syria, and my workplace experiences—not to mention my newly-gained freedom in reading materials—caused a slow, steady, and irreversible erosion in these Syrian-born convictions. I've already described my rejection of Ba'athism as a process of unlearning that was years in the making. With my residency at Henry Ford, I was embarking upon another unlearning and conversion experience, this one truly life-changing. I did not know it at the time, but the old bigoted Tarif was about to die off and a more tolerant, humane Tarif about to be born. Everything that I've written so far leads up to this conversion, and everything that I write afterward follows as its consequence.

During my first visit to American medical facilities in Minnesota, uncle Bashar and aunt Diane acted as my chaperones—so, in effect, their successes shielded me from my own self-doubts. I've already given my impression of the medical school's magnificent facilities and the hospital's efficient, collegial, cooperative staffing. During that first visit, questions of race, religion, and ethnicity never entered into my mind—possibly, because my aunt and uncle were well established and were treated with such respect. But their professional reality had yet to become my own, and I was painfully aware that I was a Syrian Muslim just beginning his career in an American hospital. My colleagues were no longer abstractions. They were going to be real people whose backgrounds were different from my own. I had grown up believing that differences in religion and ethnicity made for inequalities in the workplace. Hierarchism, factionalism, and favoritism were endemic within the Syrian version of institutionalized health care. So my expectations upon entering Henry Ford were filtered through my prior work experience. My first task would be to "learn my place" within the hierarchy. I would learn whom to trust and whom to avoid. And, generally, I'd stay out of trouble by becoming invisible. All this, of course, belonged to the Ba'athist mindset that I had yet to throw off.

What I didn't expect was the kindness that my American professors lavished on me. The program director whom I worked with, Dr Jeffrey M DeVries, was Jewish. He gave me honest guidance and support, and I wasn't an exception in this regard. He took a number of Syrian doctors into his program and under his wing. Another of my supervisors, Dr Mark Goetting, was Christian. He treated me as solicitously as he would have his own son. I was touched by the humanity of these doctors. Through their example, I was beginning to judge people "by the content of their character," as Martin Luther King, Jr, put it, rather than by their religious, racial, or ethnic background. I can quote the Reverend King now, but when I first started my residency in Detroit, I knew little about the man and his legacy. That would soon change.

While in Detroit, I spent my free time reading and renting movies, one of which was Ben Kingsley's *Gandhi*. I don't remember it showing in Damascus back when it was released in 1982. Of course I knew what Gandhi meant to post-colonial India. Being Hindu, Mohandas Karamchand "Mahatma" Gandhi was not going to be held up as a spiritual example for students in Ba'athist Syria. Neither would the Buddhist spiritual leader, the Dalai Lama, nor the Catholic Mother Theresa, nor the Black Southern Baptist preacher, Martin Luther King, Jr. I had heard of these great men and women. But I hadn't been taught much about them. I didn't know, for example, that Gandhi sought the spiritual unity of all faiths in God and that he was a friend of Christians and Muslims alike. (I've read recently that he was assassinated for being too accommodating to Muslims—that he refused to use power on behalf of India's Hindus.) Besides, my schooling in Hinduism can be stated in one sentence. A Hindu, I was taught, is a *kafir* or "idol worshipper," which violates Islam. Case closed.

But, in America, I was free to choose what I wished to read and watch and, one evening, I chose to watch *Gandhi*. I was humbled by the man's compassion, inspired by his commitment to justice, and intrigued by his practice of nonviolence. I was also struck by the parallels between Palestine under British mandate and India under British colonial rule. Had he not been felled by an assassin's bullet in 1948—the year Israel won its independence while keeping land that had been designated for a Palestinian state—I'm sure that Gandhi would have appealed for Palestinian justice, rights, and equality.

Back in Jordan, I had watched an initially nonviolent demonstration turn ugly. Still, Gandhi's commitment to nonviolent resistance was a revelation to me, so I set out to read about his life and works in such collections as *All Men Are Brothers*[15] and *The Essential Gandhi*.[16] "I object to violence," Gandhi wrote, "because when it appears to do good, the good is only temporary. The evil it does is permanent." "*Here*," I thought to myself as I read, "*is the Palestinian problem in a nutshell: no good has ever come from violence in the Middle East, even when people believe in the justice of their cause.*"

I read more: "The weak," Gandhi wrote, "can never forgive. Forgiveness is the attribute of the strong." I believed—or, rather, I wanted to believe—these words. But words like these are world-changing, and they change the meaning of other value-terms, as well. For example, not only "strength" but "courage" changes in its meaning. When you are taught that vengeance is a marker of manliness and that the failure to revenge is weakness, then Gandhi's words seem very wrong—and yet true, nonetheless.

And I read more: "Where there is love there is life." This last sentence seemed so simple on the surface, so obvious. And yet, as I contemplated its message, I realized how so many of us had been born and raised on hate, love's opposite. Certainly I had been raised on a daily dose of prejudice. I may not have been a Ba'athist, and I may not have committed crimes against the state or the people of Syria, but I would never have said that my life centered around love. Duty, yes. Religious observance, occasionally. But love? No, no.

In the midst of these meditations, one point seemed irrefutable. It was by nonviolent means that Gandhi had won rights for his people. "Had Gandhi been born in Palestine," I mused, "could his methods have brought peace—and justice—to the Middle East?"

"Yes," I was tempted to say, But . . . no, no. Gandhi's idealism might have served Hindu Indians, but Sunni Arabs? No, I couldn't see the connection to Islam. My studies in ethics and in what I have come to call the Quran of peace were only beginning.

From Gandhi, I moved on to the Mahatma's great American disciple in nonviolence, the reverend Martin Luther King, Jr. In his *Papers*,[17] Dr King writes of visiting India in 1959 to study with Gandhi's disciples: "Since being in India, I am more convinced than ever before that the method of nonviolent resistance is the most potent weapon available to oppressed people in their struggle for justice and human dignity" (13). To this day, when I listen to recordings of his great speeches, like "I Have A Dream" (1963), I am caught up by the thrilling, tremulous cadence of his voice. One doesn't have to be a native English speaker to be moved by his words.

True to the Mahatma's example, Dr King touched a nation's conscience and turned nonviolent protest into a victory for civil rights. Like Gandhi, King preached love: "Darkness cannot drive out darkness, only light can do that. Hate cannot drive out hate, only love can do that." Like Gandhi, he

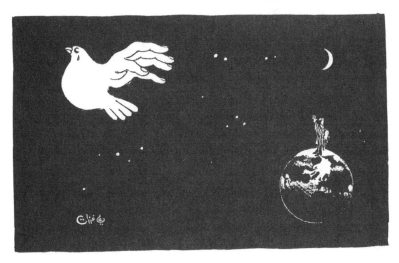

helped harness vast historical forces with his eloquence and moral stance. And, like Gandhi, he was assassinated.

My foray into ethics soon became professional as well as personal and spiritual. During my residency at Henry Ford, I learned that most important medical decisions have an ethical component and that medical practice is at heart an ethical practice. Thus began my systematic study of medical ethics— a study which I continue to this day. Having completed a Master's degree in bioethics at the University of Toronto (2006), I have taught various courses in medical ethics both in Syria and here in the States. (In a future chapter, I'll write about my teaching in Syria.) But, during those first months of study on my own, I found myself compartmentalizing aspects of my readings, my work, my beliefs, my relationships, and my life. I was as yet uncertain how it all "fit together," particularly how it all fit within Islam—or at least within the version of Islam that I had been taught and had practiced since childhood.

I have mentioned the plight of Palestinians many times in this chapter. One reason is that many of my relatives and friends in Detroit were Palestinian. At the very moment that my friends proudly, often defiantly declared themselves Palestinian, I had to admit that I no longer knew what the phrase itself, "being Palestinian," meant. I understood how the term was used historically, politically, and ethnically. I understood how it entailed certain stereotypes, even in the Arab world. I understood and sympathized with the feelings of homelessness and uprootedness, of being kicked from one job to another and from one place to another, constantly under suspicion. And I suppose I understood, though I could no longer condone, the militancy of those who sought to win their rights back by force. I was beginning to believe that there was something more definitive, more essential, more real than "being Palestinian," and that was being human.

This is what my residency at Henry Ford was teaching me. It was not their Jewishness or their Christianity, but their humanity that made my hospital supervisors into models of ethical behavior. But I still hadn't figured out how I, as a Muslim, fit into this new humanitarianism. After all, the kindness of my hospital supervisors did not negate their Jewishness or their Christian beliefs. I wanted to say that being fully human—that is, being fully humane, having grown into an ethical creature whose motives rested in compassion, peace, justice, and charity—was a precondition of being fully Jewish, fully Christian, fully Hindu, fully Buddhist.

But, when it came to be "fully Muslim," the Islamic teachings of my youth caused me to hesitate over this same, humane proposition. A Muslim (whose very name in Arabic means "one who submits to God") is to focus his thoughts on God, not on man. Though sharia law enjoins us to acts of charity, I could not yet decide whether the fullness of humanitarianism as practiced by Gandhi, King, and other men and women of peace had its roots in Islam, specifically, or in a core set of beliefs that historically have been common to the three great monotheistic religions: Islam, Christianity, and Judaism.

Until I could resolve this dilemma for myself, I could not complete, much less embrace fully, my studies in humanitarian ethics.

While living in Detroit, I did something that I would never have dreamed of doing in Syria. I attended prayers at a Shiite mosque. I had Shiite friends back in Syria, but the divide separating Shia from Sunni was never crossed without creating some sense of scandal. It's hard to imagine that two religious sects, both followers of the Prophet (peace be upon him), have built up such mutual hatred as to slit each other's throats. So I attended Shiite prayers to judge for myself whether the differences were worth dying for. After several visits, I came to the insight that, despite controversies separating Sunni from Shia, there was an essential unity in all of Islam, a unity that came from God.

But my struggles to understand continued. I knew that God demands our submission. I knew that He requires our obedience. Surely He asks for our love, as well? And does He not command us to love each other? To love ourselves? Our God is a God of justice. So much I knew. Our God is a God of mercy. This I knew, too. Is our God a God of love? I wanted to say yes, but I couldn't see much evidence in the way most of my fellow Muslims taught and practiced Islam. In my struggles, I delved further into the traditions of Islam.

It was as good as impossible for me to study Sufism while living in Syria. The Ba'athists, being secularists, had no interest in Sufi spirituality. Neither did most Sunni Imams and other intellectuals, who were content to treat the Five Pillars of Islam (*Shahadah* or declaration of faith; *Salat* or ritual prayer; *Zakat* or tithing for the poor; *Sawm* or fasting during Ramadan; and *Hajj* or pilgrimage to Mecca) legalistically rather than spiritually. What I was discovering in my study of Sufism was that the world of Islam was larger than the legalism I had been taught. There is a spiritual dimension at the heart of Islam, which draws adherents to an awareness of God's abiding presence in the here-and-nowness of one's soul-life. And I was eager to seek His presence.

I do not wish to make this chapter into a lesson in theology. I am not a theologian, after all, and the subtleties of Sufi experience lie beyond my capacities to describe or explain. The masters of Sufism—from the Prophet's disciples like Abou Bakr, Omar, Othman, and Ali to al-Qushairi, al-Junaid, and al-Hafi—have been my guides, and the best that I can do is point the reader to their texts. What I wish to do here is to describe the process of my "change of heart" with respect to war and peace—for war was the subject that precipitated this theological digression.

So: I was home from work one evening, sitting in my apartment, reading a saying by the prophet Mohammad (peace be upon him): "All creatures are the children of God and those most beloved by Him are the ones most beneficent to His children." It's not as if this particular hadith rose up off the page. Reading it wasn't a mystic experience in itself. But I felt as if its meaning "opened" like a floodgate, filling me to the brim. "*If we are all children of God,*" I thought to myself, "*then we gain God's love by showing love to all—not just to our fellow Muslims, but to all God's children.*" Then another saying opened in similar manner: "You will not be a true believer of God until you wish your brothers what you wish for your selves." Here, too, there was no distinction between Muslim and non-Muslim. All are "brothers in humanity."

And other sayings "opened." Some spoke of imitating God's mercy: "Be merciful to those on earth so the one in heaven will be merciful to you." Well, "those on earth" include Muslim and non-Muslim alike as well as all creatures and the environment at large. Some spoke against oppression: "God told the Prophet (peace upon him), 'O my servants, I have forbidden oppression for myself and have made it forbidden amongst you, so you do not oppress one another.'" And some spoke of forgiveness: "The Prophet (peace upon him) told us about a man who was going to heaven because he forgave everyone before sleeping every night."

It was this last saying that hit hardest. I knew to ask forgiveness for my own sins, but I hadn't thought of forgiving others (much less of forgiving "everyone") as a step to heaven. I understood now that true peace comes through forgiving. I've known that unforgiveness makes for sleepless nights, but I'd never thought of forgiving as a nightly task. And I understood that "everyone" means everyone, Muslim and non-Muslim alike.

As I've hinted, I have no interest in turning this chapter into a theological apology or debate. But I did find these same sentiments expressed in the holy Book of Islam, and I came to conclude that I could no longer use the Quran to justify oppression, or revenge, or war against non-Muslims:

> And good and evil are not alike. Repel evil with that which is best. And lo, he between whom and thyself was enmity will become as though he were a warm friend. But none is granted it save those who are steadfast. And none is granted it save those who possess a large share of good. (Quran 41:35-36)

When we meet evil with good, then our one-time enemy "will become as though he were a warm friend." God will see to that, so long as we prove faithful to His command. Besides, we are taught to pray "In the name of Allah, the Gracious, the Merciful." How can we expect to receive God's mercy, if we show no mercy to our "brothers in humanity"?

"Surely in the breasts of humanity is a lump of flesh, if sound then the whole body is sound, and if corrupt then the whole body is corrupt. Is it not the heart?" These are the words of the Prophet (peace be upon him), which led me to the realization that a change of mind must be preceded by a change of heart. In my case, surely, this was true. I felt compassion for my "brothers in humanity" before I understood it fully. And, once I had changed emotionally, I began to change intellectually. Before long, I had become a new Tarif— more devoted to faith than before, desirous to live in the presence of God, humbled by God's mercy, a fledgling humanitarian. Such was my experience working in Detroit and studying Islam during the First Gulf War.

6
Returning to Teach in Damascus
(Receiving a Favor from Bashar)

Abu Musa reported that the Prophet, peace be upon him, said: "Feed the hungry, visit the sick, and free the captives."

—Hadith, Fiqh us-Sunnah

When I graduated from Damascus University Medical School in 1988, I left as quickly as possible for America. Again, I was following in my paternal uncles' footsteps, as both Hisham and Bashar came to the States to continue their medical studies. I went to the Henry Ford Hospital in Detroit, Michigan, where I completed my residency in pediatrics. But, truth to tell, I had a more pressing reason for leaving Syria. Had I stayed, I would have had to follow my fellow med school graduate, Bashar, into the military. I guess that made me a Syrian "draft dodger." (Can you blame me?) My only other option was to begin post-graduate studies at Damascus University—where I had endured quite enough, thank you very much.

Throughout the 1990s, I lived the nomadic existence of an academician. Having completed my residency in 1992, I moved from Detroit to Houston, Texas, where I held a fellowship in Child Neurology at the Baylor College of Medicine. Completing the fellowship in 1995, I moved from Houston to Cleveland, Ohio, where I held a fellowship in Epilepsy at the Cleveland Clinic Foundation from 1995 to 1996. In 1996, I moved from Cleveland to Chicago, Illinois, where I held a fellowship in Movement Disorders at the Rush University Medical School. In 1997, I moved from Chicago to Boston, Massachusetts, where I held Fellowships in Neurophysiology and Behavioral Sleep Medicine at the Harvard Medical School. And, having built up my credentials, I moved back to Cleveland in 1998, where I became assistant professor of Child Neurology at Case Western Reserve University. I would spend the next four years teaching at Case Western.

In June, 2000, I took the summer off from teaching and flew to Amman,

Jordan, to visit cousins. Though a dozen years had passed since I left, I dared not return to visit friends and family in Syria, where I dodged military service. I remember sitting on my Jordanian cousin's couch on the afternoon of June 10, watching *Aljazeera*. A breaking news report declared that Syrian President Hafez al-Assad had died.

I sat speechless, unbelieving. And when it finally sank in, I thanked God that the world was at last rid of Hafez. The Syrian propaganda of my youth had seared into my head the conviction—the delusion, actually—that Hafez would be Syria's president for eternity. The news of his death delighted me, and I assumed that most Syrians shared in my joy. The strong man who had seized the nation's wealth and destroyed our education system, our judicial system, our freedom of speech was gone—at last.

Granted, he had help in raping Syria's economy and its population, having built a vast, Soviet-style apparatus of hundreds of thousands of Ba'athists whom he paid to prop up his rule. But there was hope in his successor. His successor would not be Hafez's brother, the murderous Rifaat, who was living in luxurious exile. Nor would it be Hafez's oldest son, the rugged Bassel, who died in 1994. "Hafez, the father of Bassel," is how Syrian media had taken to calling the old dictator, as if to prepare Syria for his heir-apparent. But Bassel wasn't wearing his seat belt when his car crashed, and so Syrians began looking to the mild-mannered, thoughtful, seemingly tolerant Bashar as next in line of succession. Might he be the great hope for Syria's future?

Hafez died on June 10, and Bashar was sworn in on July 17, 2000. In the interim, Syria's Constitution had to be rewritten to lower the mandatory age for the presidency from forty to thirty-five—Bashar's age at the time. Reports from Syrian friends and family—for I had returned to Cleveland—showed real promise. Social discussion clubs were opening up in and around Damascus. For the first time in modern Syria, free and open debate was being tolerated. Truly, the Syrian people had hope for President Bashar al-Assad. And I had hope.

I felt this same hope in 2001. Though I had grown comfortable living in the States, I had also grown impatient with the "publish or perish" mentality of American university teaching. As I've noted, I was teaching at Case Western at the time. And with diligence I did my research, co-authored articles, gave presentations, sat on committees, and strove to be a cooperative, productive colleague—a "team player," as they say. I loved the teaching and the time spent with patients, but I was wearying of these other, seemingly more mundane aspects of professional life. In America, the talent pool is such that no one person is indispensable. (Leave aside for the moment the fact that we do have a 30% shortage of child neurologists in the US.) If Dr Tarif Bakdash, Assistant Professor at Case Western Reserve University, dared walk out of the classroom and not return, a line would form behind him of young, enthusiastic, trained professionals, each clamoring for his job.

In Syria, as in other developing countries, the situation is far different. This I knew. In Cleveland, a trained professional may be easily replaced, but that same individual would be indispensable—virtually irreplaceable—in Damascus. With Bashar al-Assad as Syrian President, I felt a sudden expansion of possibilities. I felt that I could accomplish more, that I could *matter more* and make more of a difference, if I went back to that place which I had once left in disgust but which, I knew, *needed* me—or, at least, needed people like me.

In sum, I felt a sense of obligation to the Syrian people welling up in me, calling me back—much like my uncle Hisham must have felt. Having studied at UCLA, he felt it his duty to return. Indeed, with his American degree and AMA board certification in hand, he became Syria's first fully certified neurosurgeon. Dr Hisham Bakdash went on to establish the Department of Neurosurgery at the Damascus University Medical School, where he spent his subsequent career teaching. So, for family reasons, I can't fault *all* faculty at Damascus University. In fact, I resolved to be the second Dr Bakdash to return to Damascus, bringing the latest in American medical science.

While Syria's pro-Soviet government railed against American politics, it admired American science and technology. And I was pretty good at rationalizing, back then: Bashar did not give the orders at Hama—the sins of the father need not be visited upon the son. And I could be forgiven my own refusal to serve in his father's military. With my conscience thus salved, I resolved to write to the new Syrian president.

I knew a Syrian woman living in Cleveland (home of Case Western) who had political connections back home. So I enlisted her help. I wrote about my studies at some of America's great universities. I wrote about my aspirations for Syrian education and health care. And, of course, I wrote in praise of Bashar al-Assad's enlightened governance. I handed the letter to my Cleveland-Syrian compatriot, who promised to deliver it on my behalf.

Some weeks later, I received a phone call from Syria. Speaking in Arabic, a man informed me that the Chief of Staff of the Presidential Palace in Damascus, Mr Abou Saleem Daboul, wished to speak to me. *"Yeah, and I'm Mother Teresa!"* I recall thinking to myself, assuming the call was a joke from a friend. Then it dawned on me that this was, indeed, a serious phone call. The aide put the Chief of Staff on the line.

Mr Daboul was cordial and gracious (like a Chief of Staff for a head of state should be, I guess). He said President Assad was pleased to receive my letter and recalled how he knew me at the university. Then he asked if I was visiting Syria any time soon. I told him I was coming in October, and he gave me a phone number to call upon my arrival.

When I arrived in Syria, I phoned the Palace and was told to wait for their call on October 5. A man called early that day and said I would be picked up at my family's home in the Malki district, but he didn't tell me when. "Just stay at home and be ready," he said. I got their return call and, early in the afternoon, a Mercedes pulled up to our house. There were two people in the car. Call them aides, agents, or what-have-you, but they were the same big, hulking sort that I remembered from my youth—only they had shaved their mustaches (that part of the *machismo* look had gone out of style) and buttoned up their shirts. I got in the back seat, and they drove me to the Presidential Palace. Standing near the top of Mount Qasioun, it was not a long drive from my parents' house.

Commissioned by Bashar's father, the New Shaab—that is, "The People's Palace" in Arabic—is a massive rectilinear structure made almost entirely of marble and intended to impress. Its turreted exterior walls, its monumental front gate, its long, high-ceiling hallways, and its spacious courtyards are meant to invoke the magnificence of ancient Assyrian kings. To me, having grown accustomed to modern American architecture, the palace resembled a series of stacked stone boxes—much like a fancy, high-rise Ramada Inn. But my impression soon changed.

As we drove up to the security gate near the bottom of the mountain on the road leading up to the palace, we were waved through without having to stop. There were soldiers, security forces, and bodyguards everywhere. We drove up to the front entrance of the Palace and I was let out of the car. There was a security checkpoint inside the front doors of the palace, but, to my amazement, I was again waved past. I was escorted through a long hallway and seated in a regal room whose windows looked down upon the noble old city of Damascus. The room was appointed with the finest Damascene furniture, the wooden chairs and tables inlaid with exquisitely swirled arabesque mosaics.

As I sat waiting, I rehearsed what I would say to the president. But then, for a few grand moments, I stood, my hands clasped behind my back, king-for-a-day, surveying Damascus from a new height. I looked down upon the main square and the Four Seasons Hotel—the city's other massive, modern ziggurat of a building. I also made note of my family home and old high school, which were actually not too far down the hill.

After fifteen minutes or so, an aide came in and declared that it was time to meet the President—and here he came, Bashar al-Assad, strolling through a side door that I had not noticed. He greeted me warmly with a kiss on the cheek, as we do in the Arab world. The first thing he said was, "What happened to your beard!"

We talked about the old days. Actually, he reminded me of a time spent together that I had forgotten, when we were hungry from studying and ran out in the rain to get sandwiches. We talked about our mutual friend, Ali. And we talked about the camps we attended. It was mandatory for all university students to attend military camp for two weeks every summer. Supposedly, this was to prepare us for war against Israel. But I suspect that it really prepared us for surviving Syria's dreadful summer heat. After two weeks of swarming flies and endless, boring patriotic lectures—not to mention an open latrine and trench so noxious as to leave its users nauseated—our return to med school seemed a return to paradise.

As we talked about camps, a scene ran through my mind when an army lieutenant caught Bashar talking out of turn to another student. The lieutenant called Bashar out and was determined to make a lesson of his misbehaving. The campers were dumbfounded. Didn't the lieutenant know he was humiliating the president's son and that his own life was hanging by a thread? He made Bashar take off his boots—which were just as cheap and shoddy as everyone else's—and made the Syrian heir-apparent hop on one foot out into the desert. Then he made him crawl back on his belly. All of us kept saying, "Don't you know who . . . ?"

To this, the lieutenant replied, imperiously, "I don't care *who* he is—he *must* be *disciplined!*"

Near the end of this exquisite torture, the lieutenant *did* come to realize what he was doing to whom. Of course, no apologies, however groveling, would have bought his life back had Bashar held a grudge. But nothing happened to the lieutenant. Bashar never told on him. And I came to admire Bashar for that.

After reminiscing over old times, we turned to our aspirations for the future. In so many ways, our hopes seemed intertwined. I talked about building a stronger health care system, about teaching at the medical school and working with the Ministry of Health. He talked about improving medicine and higher education and making the nation more democratic. (You'll remember that I mentioned the social clubs that had formed, where people gathered to discuss Syria's future. While on this trip, I attended one such meeting in a large house where fifty people had gathered. I found the discussion

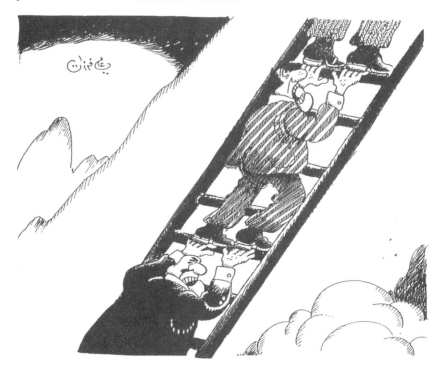

refreshingly free and open—despite the presence of *mukhabarat* (intelligence agents), who were taking mental notes. I think that, after my visit to the palace, I was willing to pretend that the *mukabarat* didn't pose a threat to the new regime's baby-steps toward freedom. I wanted to forget their presence: such was my folly at the time.)

As the president and I talked about the future, a servant brought in two demitasse cups of Arabic coffee. The cups were handsome and delicate, featuring the Presidential seal with the Syrian eagle. The pungent aroma of Arabic coffee always brings me wide awake, even before I taste it. And this coffee was like nectar of the ancient gods. Soon after the coffee was brought in, another aide came in and handed Bashar a card. The president read the card and, standing up, said, "Tarif, please excuse me, I have a phone call from the Prime Minister of Canada."

We spoke some more after he returned. Then he told his Chief of Staff, Mr Daboul, to phone the Minister of Higher Education, Dr Hassan Ryesheh, and the Minister of Health, Dr Iyad Shaati. With the polite formality of a dictator, Bashar made it known that the good doctors Ryesheh and Shaati would soon be making my acquaintance and utilizing my talents. With visions of Mercedes Benzes dancing through my head, I realized that I had just moved up more than a few rungs of the Ba'athist ladder. What I didn't appreciate was that the higher one climbs, the greater the danger of heights.

* * *

In February, 2003, I started teaching medical ethics at Damascus University Medical School to a class of 600 fifth-year students. For the professors at the medical school who had taught the course before me, the subject of bioethics was mostly about medical "bedside manners" and the history of Islamic medicine. Despite my years of experience after completing medical school there in Damascus, despite having completed fellowships at Baylor College of Medicine, the Cleveland Clinic, Rush University Medical School, and Harvard Medical School, and despite having taught as assistant professor at Case Western Reserve University Medical School, I was now under contract as a Syrian government employee receiving a paycheck of $150 a month.

I knew that the class would reflect Syria's ethnic and religious diversity. My students, though Sunni predominantly, would include Shiites and Alawites, Christians (both Orthodox and Catholic), Ismaili, and Druze. As I stepped up to the long wooden table that separated me from the students, I surveyed the same old auditorium where I had taken medical classes some twenty years before. Nothing had changed in that time, not even that table or the uncomfortable wooden seats in the auditorium, (Well, I suppose they had changed somewhat, being twenty years older. For that matter, I too had changed over those twenty years.) The room looked like a Greek amphitheater, and I, the protagonist, the main actor, had just taken the stage.

High on the wall to my right was the same glassed picture frame with a portrait of the Syrian president. When I sat as a student it was the image of Hafez al-Assad glaring down on proceedings. Here it was his son Bashar—the man who helped put the dry-erase marker in my hand. (They used chalk and a blackboard back in my days at med school, so this at least was an improvement.) But it was the same cranky old microphone from twenty years ago that I bent to turn on.

I recalled sitting in this same room when a short, a mustached cardiologist ended his lecture with the declaration, "Now, if anyone has a question, he must be a donkey." Not waiting to see if there were any of that "ignoramus" species in the room, he turned and left. I was determined not to be that guy. Rather than shut down students' questioning, I would teach in the Socratic method, by the intellectually-democratic two-way-street of dialogue.

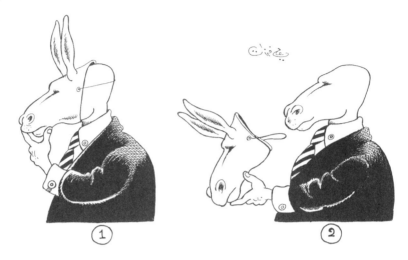

So, after a brief introduction, I began with a series of questions that caught students off guard.

"Did any of you choose your parents?" I asked. They shook their heads in unison, and said, puzzled, "No."

"Did any of you choose the city you were born in?" This time they replied in confident chorus, "No!"

"*This class is going to be a breeze,*" I can imagine them thinking. Their fears about this new teacher and the subject of bioethics had been unfounded.

"Did any of you choose your religion?" That gave them a moment of pause, though one young woman replied, confidently, "Yes, I chose the religion *of my parents.*" But the other 600 or so students seemed to hesitate over her answer.

"Do any of you deserve to be hated, hurt, discriminated against, or condescended to because of the parents who bore you, the city you were born in, or the religion you practice?"

They replied "no," but with less confidence. I glanced at one athletic-looking young man sitting in the front row wearing an un-pressed white button-up shirt and khaki trousers. He looked like he'd just been slapped in the face. I wanted to ask him, "What are you thinking?" But I didn't want to interrupt his train-of-thought. It was likely a train he was boarding for the first time, and he didn't yet know where it was going to take him.

Then I said, "Look closely at the student to your left and the student to your right." With a sweeping gesture of my right hand, I added, "Look around the auditorium at all your fellow students." They were starting to squirm by this time.

Then I asked them (and they could see this coming), "Do you have the right to hate any people in this room because of their parents, or the city where they were born, or their religion?" By this time, I noticed a lot of face twitching, shoulder jerking, and other involuntary physical movement. The students couldn't say no, but they weren't ready to say yes. I watched as twenty-two years of certitude melted into confusion on their faces.

I allowed the class to suffer a few moments of silence (punctured by an occasional, awkward shuffling of hands and feet) in contemplation of this last question. And I was not unaffected by my own question. I, too, was reliving the rage I felt as a teenager for what the Israelis had done to my mother, for what they had done in Lebanon, driving the PLO to the sea and Arafat into exile—for the deaths of thousands along the way, all by superior Israeli airpower and high-powered artillery and arrogance. The choking tightness in my chest brought back the humiliation I felt back then, when I was a student in Syria. It was a feeling that Israel would always have its way with Syria and with all its Arab neighbors. And yet, as I stood there working through my own emotions, I reminded myself that Arafat killed innocent Israelis. It was the assassination of Israeli athletes at the 1972 Munich Games that brought misfortune to my family. I can blame the Israeli Mossad, but I can't excuse or exempt Arafat's Black September.

When I was twenty-two—the age of most of the students sitting before me then—I felt overwhelmed by anger toward Israel. But my feelings toward Ba'athist Syria weren't much better. As to my own government, I felt a sense of powerlessness and a pervasive anxiety bordering on fear. This ambivalence had been building throughout high school, but it came to a head in 1982, when I was beginning college.

Even as the Israelis were hunting down Arafat's PLO, General Rifaat al-Assad (President's Hafez al-Assad's brother) was slaughtering thousands of Syrians—men, women, and children—in the Hama Massacre. His target was the Muslim Brotherhood, but his victims were all Sunni Muslims, just like me. That made me feel personally vulnerable, to say the least. The lesson I took from the Hama massacre of 1982 was that, in Assad's Syria, they could do anything they wanted to anyone they wanted to do it to, at any time they wanted. And that "anyone" could be a teenaged student at Al-Thaqafi School in Damascus—or a teacher of bioethics at the Damascus University Medical School.

After we got past that first battery of questions, a sigh of relief seemed to pass through the auditorium. We *could* talk, frankly and freely, about culturally sensitive and even seemingly "dangerous" topics without being punished. It was as if the students in that room had been holding their breath for many,

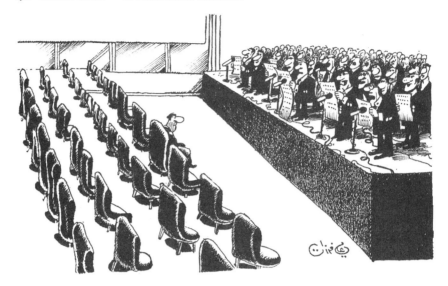

many years. After discussing inherited belief systems back and forth for some time, I began my next set of questions.

"Are human beings or animals more ethical?"

"Human beings," they answered, "of course."

"So, do animals of the same species fight each other to the death? Do they organize into enemy camps and fight wars?"

"No, of course not," was their reply.

"Now, if we humans are so moral, why would we ever refuse to help people who are sick or starving and can't help themselves?" They gave no answers, although I could see each question working its way into their psyches.

I continued my intellectual assault: "At the core of the oath that you will take as a Muslim physician," I reminded these med students, "is the ideal not only to heal patients following best medical practice, but *never to do harm to anyone*. And that's a good place to start a discussion of bioethics. How can you be entrusted to heal someone you don't respect, whom you don't treat as an equal, whom you don't value as fellow human being?"

Ironically, when I sat in this auditorium as a medical student, the question of bioethics—or of ethics of any kind, really—didn't enter my mind. I was either too busy or too distracted by the demands of daily life and studies. And I wasn't alone. Ethical questions of the sort I was asking were not part of our lives back then—at least not in a direct, open, conscious way, either at home or at school.

My strategy on that first day of class was to break the old patterns of expectation, to open minds, to raise up the students' comfort levels and get them used to asking, and answering, moral questions. For the most part, they had grown up being taught to obey and *not* ask questions, so this was a whole new journey for most. We needed to set off slowly at first, since we were tiptoeing toward a minefield—which is how I'd describe the state of medical ethics in Syria in 2003.

After that first class, students from other programs started coming—from English Literature, Business, and Information Technology, to name several. Apparently, word had spread of our grand experiment in academic freedom. Many came out of a sense of curiosity, wondering what an intellectual "open forum" looked and sounded like. Some sat back and listened. Others joined in. And while the discussions became heated at times, they remained civil— for the ground rules were pretty simple. To have a right to speak, you had to wait your turn and listen. You had to avoid personal insult. And you had to mean what you said.

I remember times when a Communist or an atheist would be in vigorous debate with a veiled woman or a bearded man without mustache (a sign of the most devout).

"Why should government or business or religion rule every aspect of our lives?"

"But if you would obey God . . ."

Students who would never have talked to each other outside of class found themselves discussing real philosophical, ethical, and bioethical subjects— and they were taking each other seriously. I wish I had thought to ask them to shake hands before or after their debates. More than symbolic, a handshake between opponents of any sort—intellectual, theological, political, what- have-you—is an acknowledgement of each person's common humanity.

As I've noted, my own med school training had nothing to do with ethics of any sort. But when I graduated from Damascus University Medical School and went off to study in America, *that's* when my immersion in ethics began.

I was twenty-four when I began my residency at the Henry Ford Hospital in Detroit. I remember being introduced to the program director—Dr DeVries, my teacher and future mentor—and shaking his hand. It was then that I noticed he was wearing a yarmulke. I had never shaken hands with a Jew before. In fact, I had never talked to a Jew before or been introduced to one. Surely *he* knew that I was Syrian and a Muslim. But, smiling, he looked me in the eye and extended his hand, welcoming me to the hospital. His smil- ing welcome confused me, though I tried to hide my confusion.

I now know that confusion is a first step in "unlearning" the prejudices of one's upbringing. That's actually what I was aiming at with those first questions in that first bioethics class in Damascus—to confuse my students in ways that would lead them to think on their own, for themselves.

From Detroit I went to Houston, where I began a residency at the Baylor College of Medicine. When I was introduced to my Department Chair at Baylor, Dr Marvin Fishman, I had my second chance, as it were, to get the introduction right. I held out my hand, smiled, and looked my new mentor in the eye. Dr Fishman was especially kind to me, as was the rest of the department. I felt welcome at Baylor, just as I was made to feel welcome at Henry Ford. It didn't matter that my teachers and mentors were Jewish or Christian while I was Muslim. I can say, gratefully, that I've never met with prejudice of any sort on a professional level while working in America. And this fact challenged me to give up my own religious prejudices.

I was aided in this personal transformation by texts that were new to me back then. The teachings of Mahatma Gandhi and Martin Luther King, Jr were unavailable to me in Syria. In America, I pored over their writings and the writings of other great men and women who had walked the path of justice and equality and peace. And then, God be praised, I was given insight into the Quran of peace by my study of Sufism. This subject—my conversion from a Muslim who lived "under the law" into a Muslim who sought to live in God's loving presence and mercy—belongs to a previous chapter. But let me state that I've always found it a delicious irony that I came, not simply to Islam, but to the *true* Islam by leaving the Arab Middle East. For it was here in America that I learned to live in accordance with the Quran of peace.

I make this point here, since my teaching of bioethics in Damascus was grounded in insights I had gained while living, studying, working, and teaching in the United States.

During that first term of teaching at Damascus University, classroom discussions were lively. But students were puzzled that I hadn't required a textbook: "How can we take a test if there's no textbook?" That was a fair question. Most tests given at Damascus University (as in universities throughout Syria) were multiple-choice. Professors tended to reuse parts of the same tests semester after semester. So, of course, students got copies of the old tests and memorized them. But the sort of textbook that I wanted to use was unavailable in Assad's Syria.

It was a rule that all courses at all Syrian universities would have a required textbook, and that this textbook be written in Arabic. These books had to be approved by the Supreme Council for Science of the Ministry of Higher Education, and I assume the reader knows what happens when politics meddles with education. The Ba'athist-approved textbooks were out of date and, assuming that they were originally in English or French, they were usually very poorly translated by professors who had been trained in the Eastern Bloc. And, if not by the professors, they were translated by the professors' poor students.

The "Arabic only" rule was ostensibly to promote Syrian nationalism. Its real effect was to limit Syrian students' access to diverse texts and, hence, to knowledge of the world outside Ba'athism. Political, ethical, social, and even scientific free-thinking posed a danger to the regime, which responded with policies of censorship and even book-banning. The consequence to Syrian medicine (and the sciences generally) was catastrophic, in that instruction was never up-to-date.

In case the reader thinks I exaggerate, I offer the following quotation from a web-based article, "Faculty of Medicine at Damascus University."[18] Given the anonymous, open-sourced nature of wiki articles, I assume the page (last modified October 4, 2014) is written and maintained by Syrian nationals who tow the Ba'ath party line:

> The College of Medicine adopts a strategy of scientific research by the Ministry of Higher Education in cooperation with various governmental bodies. Contributing members of the faculty in the College of Medicine are an important part of science activities as established annually by the Supreme Council for Science of the Ministry of Higher Education. The research presented in the course of medical researchers, as well as new faculty members[,] are allowed access to translated research acquired through doctorates from the university to the Arab world. This translation is provided with identity cards required with faculty membership. This is important in the Arabization of science and research: It is believed research in the mother tongue should be accessible to a large segment of beneficiaries.

There's no need "to read between the lines" here. In every respect, the free pursuit of medical science has been coopted by party politics. The article's authors openly declare that government-issued "identity cards" are required for access to research, that research subjects are planned "in cooperation with various government bodies" (for which, read "the Ba'ath Party"), and that any research made available to any student or faculty member must first be translated into Arabic.

I would have none of that. In preparing for class discussion, I used the fifth edition of Winslade, Siegler, and Jonsen's *Clinical Ethics*.[19] Needless to say, there was no chance that the Supreme Council for Science of the Ministry of Higher Education would approve an American textbook for classroom use. And even if the Supreme Council approved it, I would have had to wait for its "Arabization," which would entail a poorly rendered and censored translation.

So, as I've noted, I didn't assign a textbook. Instead, I based my tests on class discussion: "What does 'ethics' mean?" "What does 'morality' mean?" "If you work in a hospital with two respirators and have three patients who will die without use of a respirator, how will you decide which patients to save?" "If a woman is raped and has conceived, is it ethical to give her a medical abortion?" "Are there ethical considerations in treating AIDS patients?"

I included this last question, since more than a few students believed that AIDS patients were likely gay, that being gay was sinful and, therefore, that AIDS patients didn't deserve treatment. "But as physicians," I reminded them, "we are not placed as judges over our patients. Besides, under Islamic law, we have a duty to treat anyone who needs our help—and, yes, that includes an Israeli, even an Israeli soldier." Even toward the end of a semester's worth of ethical discussion, that last statement was still jolting to many students.

At the end of one of my classes, after I had been teaching for two years at Damascus, a student came up to my desk. Apparently, she was concerned about an upcoming exam.

"Professor," she said, "I heard your questions need thinking to answer."

I replied, smiling, "My dear, what questions *don't* need thinking to answer?"

Most of my students did do well. Most appreciated being able to express their thoughts and being heard with respect—something that many had never experienced before in a public forum.

Each year, on the last day of class, I would wish them all the best and remind them, "Be compassionate to all." And every year they would applaud me as the class ended. I always had tears in my eyes on that last day, for their applause surrounded me with feelings of love.

In 2004—my last year of teaching at Damascus—I asked a friend who was an accomplished violinist to come play Schubert's *Ave Maria*. It's ironic that my friend, who is an atheist, was going to play a piece of Christian music written by a German composer to a Syrian class of predominately Muslim medical students, most of whom had never heard Schubert—much less heard a classical violinist playing live. In some Muslim traditions, music of any sort is forbidden, so I was neither surprised nor offended when several students left. Those who remained sat quietly, as if in a meditative state.

Since middle school, I've loved classical music. I've made this point several times already. I've never practiced "music therapy" consciously, though I've played soft music in my medical offices and in my private clinic. I've felt its calming effects myself, and I believe I've seen it calm and caress my patients, the young ones especially. Still you might ask, why invite a violinist to a class in bioethics? I think that music, like morality, makes its appeal to our common humanity. I can't imagine anyone listening well to Schubert's musical prayer and not feeling lifted up and enlarged. Those who *feel* more will have more empathy and will serve patients better. Hence, music is itself a medicine for the soul.

As I've noted, most of my students had never heard a Western classical violinist. Those who were in school by merit as opposed to cronyism—like the parachuters of my old med school class—were intelligent and hard-working. And many, if not most, were from poor families. Here they were, among the top baccalaureate students in Syria, and yet they were surviving day-to-day, meal-to-meal, and class-to-class. As I write, I can see their faces still. Entranced by Schubert, they seem to have laid their cares aside, if only for a few moments, to dream of a bright, fulfilling future.

And yet, as I conclude this chapter—a little more than eleven years after that semester's first classroom discussion—I admit to have wondered if my lessons were "too little, too late" for those students and for my country. If the 600 students in that first bioethics class are taken as a microcosm of war-torn Syria today, then many will have left to practice medicine in the EU or the States. Of those that remain, as many as half will now be living and working in refugee camps. Some others will have died. Some others will be in prison even as the reader reads this sentence. Some will be maimed and some will be facing torture, because of the civil war—and all because of who their parents were, what city they were born in, and what religion they were given as a precious gift and birthright.

7
Working with the First Lady
(I Become Syria's Secretary General for the Disabled)

And of people there are some who say, "we believe in Allah and the last day," but they really do not believe. They seek to deceive Allah and those who have faith, but they deceive none but themselves, and they are not aware. In their hearts is a disease, so Allah has increased their disease and there awaits them a painful punishment . . . And when it is said to them, "do not make corruption on earth," they say, "verily, we are only reformers." Indeed, they themselves are the corruptors, but they are not aware.

—Quran 2:8-12

Syrian-born, the daughter of affluent parents, Asma Akhras grew up in the United Kingdom and attended King's College, London, graduating in 1996 with degree emphases in computer science and French. Bashar al-Assad had himself studied in England, where the two met. He was unmarried in July, 2000, when he became Syrian leader. But every Syrian leader needs a wife, so he was quickly cured of his bachelorhood. His father Hafez died in June; Bashar was made President in July; Asma Akhras returned to Syria in November. She married and became Asma al-Assad in December. Was her marriage an affair of the heart or an affair of state? At the time, such a question seemed irrelevant, since Asma offered us so much hope.

For the most part, Syrians welcomed and embraced their new First Lady. Glamorous indeed, highly cultured, well educated, passionately committed to progressive causes. These were qualities that England's Princess Diana possessed in her lifetime. More than a nation, the world came to trust and admire, even love Lady Di. Raised in the UK and taught by Lady Di's example, Asma was now Syria's own. If she possessed even a fraction of the charisma and commitment of her English role model, then Asma's causes could become the Syrian nation's causes. We had reason, indeed, to hope back then.

Lady Di's untimely death brought no celebrations in the Middle East. For the time that she was married to Prince Charles, she helped raise his popularity worldwide—though, in truth, she became far more popular than her husband, because she was more sympathetic, more accessible, more *visible* than the seemingly aloof Prince of Wales. And she was unafraid of risk-taking. How can anyone working in health care forget that moment when Lady Di reached out and shook the hand of an AIDS patient, proving to the world that HIV was not communicable by casual contact? Few heads of state would have shown the same courage as this young woman and mother—and princess, though the title didn't seem to have seduced her. She used the charisma accruing to royalty, but not for selfish gains. Rather, she combined her own native charm with the aura of royalty in pursuit of charitable works. Lady Di was kindhearted. She was smart. And she was fierce in support of the poor, the sick, and the downtrodden.

The Syrian First Lady, Asma Assad was fourteen years younger than the Princess of Wales, yet they both seemed to promise ordinary citizens that government could raise itself to match the highest sentiments of its people. The two women were powerful, yet fragile. Lady Di was lost in the violence of a Paris car wreck. Asma Assad lives on, but her effectiveness was lost in the violence of Dara'a, the first siege of the Syrian civil war.

A great surge of hope ran through Syria when Bashar became President in 2000. Truth to tell, I found my hopes increased by First Lady Asma who married Bashar later the same year. Through the first decade of the twenty-first century, *she* was the face of reform in Syria, championing women's rights, Westernized education, and progressive health care (among other noble causes). And, for the latter half of this decade, I worked with her on elements of this reform.

In 2001, I wrote my fateful letter to President Assad, offering to return to teach. And, after phone calls by the Palace Chief of Staff, I was teaching the next year at the Damascus University Medical School, hoping to bring change to Syrian education in health care. But I soon learned that it was not medical technology or medical science that was most lacking. What Syrian health care lacked most egregiously was a system of ethics. Paying mere lip service to the Syrian Physician's Oath, Syria's doctors (not all, but many—too many) had become servants of the Ba'ath Party and not of the people. Faced with that insight, I needed to make myself into someone capable of teaching, not medicine simply, but medical ethics. And I knew that medical ethics rested on a broader, philosophical foundation of ethics generally.

Medical ethics apparently was a problem facing health care systems throughout the Arab Middle East, and I was not the first person to notice it. In 2004, I was appointed the Academic Coordinator for the World Health Organization of the United Nations in Damascus. The World Health Organization (WHO) had just established a grants program whereby physicians would be hand-picked and sent to the University of Toronto to study ethics. I was selected and, in 2005, I left for Toronto, Canada, to begin a master's degree in applied ethics. Covering tuition and fees and a stipend, WHO gave me a "free ride," as they say in the States. Let me take this opportunity to thank WHO and other United Nations organizations for the good that they have done over the years for people and nations such as my own.

I finished the degree in 2006 and came back to Syria with the intention of "applying the ethics" that I had learned. But I felt strangely unsettled. I hadn't found my niche professionally and I didn't know where I would find it. I hadn't found it at Damascus University and I didn't know where else to look. And then, in the midst of my restlessness, I received a phone call from a Saudi friend who had trained at Case Western while I was teaching there. He asked if I'd be interested in a one-month *locum* residency teaching physicians in Riyadh, the Saudi capital.

"Yes," I told him: "I'd love to—you caught me at the perfect time."

The Saudi Kingdom enjoys the best health care system in the Middle East. That's according to the World Health Organization, and I saw nothing to contradict that assertion. Financed by the nation's oil wealth, the facilities at Riyadh's King Fahd Medical City—indeed, it was big enough to be named a city-within-the-city—were top-flight. And my personal accommodations were grand. I felt treated like a Saudi prince—up to a point, of course. I stayed in my own private villa. And the pay by any measure, Syrian or American, was regal.

The month of my residency soon passed and I was heading back to Syria. I had enjoyed the Saudi medical staff personally and professionally. And I was well-liked and well-respected. So much so, that the hospital administration offered to hire me permanently. It was a tempting offer in many ways: fabulous pay, fabulous accommodations, fabulous benefits and vacation time. So I left for Damascus and waited for the paperwork to arrive. A career in the fabled Kingdom seemed just over the horizon.

The employment application arrived, and I sat down with it, pen in hand. But I couldn't bring myself to complete it. There was a restlessness in me, still. In Syria, I felt at home culturally but not yet professionally. In the Saudi Kingdom, I felt at home professionally but not culturally. The King Fahd Medical City was grand, but I found life in the city of Riyadh suffocating—stifling in almost every respect.

In Syria, the First Lady can be seen and photographed unveiled. The nation's imams might grouse, but she shares that freedom and right with other Syrian women (though again, it's a freedom that ISIS threatens to take away). Now, for readers unfamiliar with life in Saudi Arabia, there is no such freedom. While Saudi princess Ameera Al-Taweelf Asma has the verve to go unveiled in public, she proves an exceedingly rare exception to the cultural rule. Almost universally, Saudi women are veiled in public. The Kingdom's morality laws are strict, sexist, and rigorously enforced—not as violently as in the Islamic State, but they are enforced nonetheless.

There was no discernible night life. There were virtually no public entertainments. I would walk the polished marble streets of Riyadh in utter boredom. Literally, there was nothing for me to do, so I spent most of my leisure time alone in my private villa. Fortunately, my Saudi friend had a few DVDs to lend me. I watched, and re-watched, episodes of *The Office* and *The Lord of the Rings*.

For days, the application for Saudi employment lay on my dinner table, half finished. I thought back to my time at Damascus University, where I was both student and teacher. Though men outnumbered women, still there were women in the same classrooms hearing the same lectures and preparing for the same professions. And then I remembered the story of a man who taught at a women's university in Riyadh. There weren't many male professors there, given the rules of segregation by gender. (Even public restaurants were segregated.) So he lectured his senior-level class of female students while standing behind a sturdy glass barrier. And when a young woman had questions, she would telephone him—during class. Class discussion would be conducted by telephone. Stories like this defy belief.

Though tempted by the luxury and prestige, I wanted, even back then, to live in a land where the Quran of peace is preached over the distorted Quran of legalism and extremism. Where modesty is a matter of conscience, not compulsion. Where tolerance reigns. And where justice is tempered with equity and, indeed, with mercy. That land was not Assad's Syria—not yet. But I was also sure that, if such a land existed, its name was not Saudi Arabia.

Though still struggling with the decision, I had managed to finish the paperwork. And that's when I visited the non-government Syrian Organization for the Disabled. Founded in 2002 by First Lady Asma, its Arabic name was AAMAL, meaning "hopes." I met with the AAMAL Executive Director—I'll call her HM—who was pleasant and showed real interest in my professional background. She asked about my plans for the future. I told her about my frustrations teaching in Syria and that I had been offered a job in Saudi Arabia.

Somewhat boldly, she asked if I'd consider working at AAMAL. There was a position opening up—the Director of Services, which supervised the clinic staff. "You should apply," she said: "After all, you have the expertise and the credentials." She was refreshingly familiar in her manner. And, even as she was commiserating over my experiences teaching, an inspiration seemed to come upon her.

"Tell you what," she said, as if setting the hook to reel me in. "We have a gala dinner coming up. Why don't you come? The First Lady is very passionate about helping the disabled. She'll be at the gala, and I'll introduce you to her."

From the beginning of our conversation, it was clear that HM was well-connected. This last offer sealed the deal. "I'd be pleased and honored to attend," was my surprisingly heart-felt response. Since her marriage to Bashar, I had admired Asma al-Assad from afar. And now I would get to meet the First Lady, face-to-face.

Back then, I owned two suits and an American St Jude Hospital tie. So I put on my St Jude tie and the better of my two suits and went off to the gala. And the Director, as she had promised, introduced me to the First Lady. Asma al-Assad was tall in her high heels, very elegant, very charming. I was on my best behavior, of course, but our conversation was easy and comfortable. There was no awkwardness on my part, no pretentiousness on her part. I had been introduced to her as a physician, a professor, and an old college friend of her husband's, but her interests lay in what I knew, not whom I knew. I told her about the favor President Assad had done in arranging for my teaching appointment. I told her about my qualifications as a pediatric neurologist specializing in the treatment of autism. I told her about my recent residency in the Saudi Kingdom. And I told her about the job awaiting me in Riyadh.

"Oh, you mustn't leave for Saudi Arabia," she said. "We need you here, especially at AAMAL. The disabled of Syria need your expertise—they need your help." Bowing, I thanked her for the confidence she placed in me. Her attention was soon drawn elsewhere and I spent the rest of the evening in a reverie, mentally "replaying the tape" of our conversation.

A few days later, I received a phone call from a board member of AAMAL. To preserve his anonymity, I'll call him TD. As I soon discovered, he was a fellow graduate of the Damascus University Medical School. But he had also earned a PhD in computer science—one of Asma's academic interests—and had worked at Microsoft in Seattle, Washington. This impressed me in more ways than one. Not only was he an intellectual, but his appointment to the AAMAL board had apparently been for merit and not mere Ba'athist loyalty.

And I knew TD to be a devout Muslim. If an unveiled and Euro-fashionable Asma could earn his respect and cooperation, then surely she could work across the spectrum of Syrian society.

TD spoke on Asma's behalf. "The First Lady," he said, "really wants you to work for AAMAL." (The words that I've just written don't convey the full force of his Arabic, which implied, "You know this is an offer you're not allowed to refuse.")

I told him about my contract in Saudi Arabia. And, in a sudden outpouring of candor, I admitted to him something that I had, for so long, tried to conceal from myself. I wanted to teach—but not in the lecture halls of Damascus University. Teaching hands-on by the bedsides of young patients, doing the daily rounds with interns at the Children's Hospital. That's what I loved doing. Meeting my words with an equal candor, his answer surprised me.

"Look, Damascus University is hopeless, it's dead," he said. "So don't waste your time there. If you want a better use of your talents and training, come work for AAMAL."

I interviewed with TD and two other board members whom I knew from medical school. If AAMAL proved true to its humanitarian ideal, if it attracted such talented, dedicated scientists like TD, if it drew support from the highest levels of the regime, then here—if anywhere in Assad's Syria—one person might make a palpable difference.

"I'll be taking a deep pay cut," I said sighing and half-jokingly, thinking of the Saudi contract, "but I accept the offer."

And so my work with the Syrian Organization for the Disabled began. I was tasked with overseeing some of Syria's top specialists in the diagnosis and treatment of speech, hearing, visual, physical, and cognitive impairment. With the First Lady's patronage, AAMAL had assembled a cadre of specialists who would serve the country's disabled. But, in accepting the position, I had made assumptions about the level of dedication its specialists "in the trenches" would be bringing to their work. The AAMAL board members were men and women of conviction. I would find out soon enough the mettle of those who were placed under me.

For so long in my studies and work, I had stood on the lower rungs of one or other ladder within Ba'athist Syria. And the problems that I faced always seemed to come top-down, from the upper rungs. As the newly-appointed Services Director for AAMAL, I was now standing nearer the top. Only, the problems were *not* coming from the top rungs—they were coming from the bottom-up. This phenomenon did more than frustrate me. It surprised me.

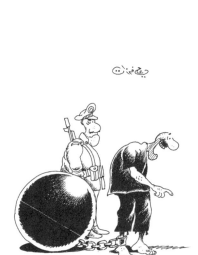
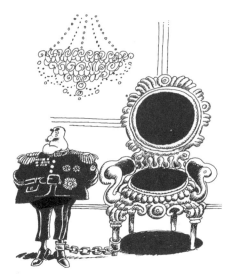

It made the problems endemic in Ba'athist hierarchy seem even more complex—and more insuperable—than I had imagined.

Most of the specialists under my supervision took their work for AAMAL as a privilege—just a paying job—rather than an opportunity to serve. Incredibly, many seemed to resent putting their talents to work for disabled children. "They're *disabled*," was a typical grouse, spoken under one's breath. Why even work for AAMAL, if you lack compassion?

It was time to put my degree in bioethics, freshly completed from the University of Toronto, to work. *This* is why I had gotten the degree to begin with. And *this* is why my work at AAMAL seemed fated.

"Listen," I'd say to one after another of my charges, "working with disabled children isn't the sort of job where you punch the time clock when you arrive and punch it again at the end of the day. Improving the lives of children with physical and mental disabilities is back-breaking, time-intensive, highly skilled labor. Everything that you've learned and trained for: *bring it and give it to these children*. No one else can help them but you. The children of Syria need you." I found myself repeating sentiments that the First Lady had spoken to me. I had found her convincing. How could one *not* be convinced, inspired even, by such sentiments?

I soon found out that exhortation, however impassioned, makes little headway against the militant indifference of Syria's specialists. The system of rewards had become so ingrained in their thinking that conscience was shoved aside, to be replaced by an all-consuming, self-justifying sense of self-entitlement.

Here was the typical mindset. Being the nation's cream-of-the-crop, they felt that they were entitled to work fewer hours in the day, not more. They felt that they were entitled to more money for less service. They felt that further training was irrelevant. I could call a meeting to discuss the latest trends in Western treatments, but their sense of militant indifference carried over from the examination room to the meeting room. While the latest in medical and physical therapies left them bored, the very notion of psychology (and of psychological therapies) left them downright indignant. At times they displayed a lack of empathy toward their young, suffering patients that spoke volumes to me. Here were men (and some women) with a more than a modicum of training, talent, and intelligence. And yet, most seemed to have had their hearts carved out and disposed of as so much Ba'athist medical waste.

I wasn't the only administrator to notice their lack of effort and militant sense of entitlement. One day, the Head of Human Resources issued a memorandum regarding workloads and hours. Of course, I agreed with its directives. But, from my perspective now, I can see why the memo was doomed from the start. Written by a non-physician to medical specialists, its impersonal, imperious tone offended our "elite team" to the core. A little more diplomacy may have enabled some give-and-take. Something middle ground might have been reachable. But the specialists reacted as a group by staging a "walk out." In effect, they went on strike, *which was unheard of in Assad's Syria.*

In response, I called a staff meeting to which they came, not in obedience so much as in curiosity as to what I'd say. Drawing on my summer-camp experiences with Syrian drill-sergeants, I raised my rhetoric up to the level of threat. "The government *will not* take this kindly," I began. "*Where* do you *think* you *are*: Switzerland?" (Sometimes things come out of my mouth that surprise even me. I was in that territory now, trying to "talk Ba'athist" as best I could.) And the fact is that the government *did* take notice and sent two tough-guy representatives over, one from the Ministry of Labor, one from Social Affairs. And what I had intimated, they declared flat out. If the specialists didn't get back to work, they'd be thrown in jail.

I had gone to AAMAL to escape Ba'athist politics and found myself standing with government agents by my side, threatening my colleagues in health care with prison. The very irony of it struck me as surreal, Kafkaesque.

It was actually the First Lady who came to the rescue, sending a close friend of hers to mediate. I'll call him AS, and I have to admit that his diplomatic skills impressed me. He managed to absorb the anger of the striking physicians while mollifying the government agents.

The crisis ended, *but nothing had changed.* Most of the specialists simply resumed their old habits. And now I had to confront the consequence of my failure. It's not that I "lost face" by failing to change the reigning culture of indifference. It's that I was *losing faith* in the power of moral exhortation. You can't impart a sense of ethics where self-interest, a sense of entitlement, and militant indifference have become institutionalized. All you can do is hold fast to your personal values, make do with the resources at hand, and make alliances with those few colleagues who share your commitments.

"*What* AAMAL *needs,*" I said to myself one frustrated morning, "*is a code of ethics.*" The specialists under my charge weren't just refusing to work, they refused to work *together.* Members of the AAMAL administration worked, ate, and socialized together. There were no sectarian, ethnic, economic, or social barriers separating us, though we were a diverse group—a mirror of Syrian society, in fact. What bound us together was our passionate commitment to a common cause. The specialists, in contrast, segregated themselves by religion and ethnicity. So I brought my idea before the Board of Trustees.

"What AAMAL needs," I said to the Board, with First Lady Asma in attendance, "is a code of ethics." I had done my homework and drafted a policy based on The United Nations Code of Ethics for Non-Profit Organizations, though modified to fit our cultural and clinical environment. With the First Lady's endorsement, my proposal was immediately adopted—only to find itself resting forevermore in a filing cabinet.

I had written an ethics code but had no means to enforce it. I knew that the specialists would resist, but I also knew that they didn't have to agree with it—at least, not at first. It's a basic rule of psychology that if you change the way a person *acts*, you can eventually change the way that person *thinks and feels.* That's what I was hoping to achieve with the specialists under my charge. (By the way, I'm aware of the irony in trying *to compel* someone to act ethically. I was beginning to feel more like a policeman and less like an administrator.)

In time, I learned that codes of ethics could work only where a beating human heart still carried the capacity for empathy, self-reflection, and a sense of personal responsibility. I had futilely encouraged, urged, and cajoled all these specialists into caring about their patients—or, at the very least, into putting in a full day's work.

And *there were* some specialists at AAMAL devoted to their work. Together, we formed a small but dedicated team. And we managed to do great good for many of the children whom God had entrusted to us. Let me state, humbly, that it was an honor to serve with those few on behalf of those many.

As AAMAL Services Director, I did have some administrative successes. While under my directorship, it remained Syria's one non-profit organization dedicated to children with visual, hearing, and autism-related conditions. AAMAL enjoyed broad support among the highest levels of the Ba'athist elite, but that was due to the Syrian First Lady, Asma al-Assad. What *she* supported, the highest echelons of society supported as a matter of course. And the organization's biggest donor was the New Shaab Palace—that is, the First Lady herself.

The Palace sponsored and paid to train "a second generation" of specialists that, in time, would replace the old corps that had revolted under my directorship. It was a slow process, one requiring foresight and considerable groundwork. As each member of the medical "old guard" retired or left, a replacement would be hand-picked and sent back to school for a graduate degree in some field pertinent to the treatment of childhood disabilities—with expenses paid by the Palace.

Again, though a slow process, this was an enlightened approach to fixing agencies like AAMAL. By educating—or re-educating—its staff, a more efficient, more *ethical* work force would take shape. I cannot stress this last point too forcefully. If we call Ba'athism a chronic social-political illness, then I'm willing to declare my own generation of Syrian physicians beyond cure. We are, in the main, a bunch of old Ba'athist dogs and, as they say, "you can't teach an old dog new tricks." Still, I can hope that the next generation—or the second, or the third generation after mine—can be educated in a better way.

(This process of education, which takes a living generation or more to complete, holds the cure for more than Syrian health care. If you ask me, "What's the single viable solution to the problems facing the Middle East today?" my answer comes in one word: "Education." For *there is no military solution* to the complex crisis that is the Middle East today. *There is no political solution* to the complex crisis that is the Middle East today. In time, there *will* be a change of heart—a change within the heart *of Islam*—that will remake the Middle East and resonate outward, teaching justice, mercy, and peace to the rest of nations on this blessed earth. But that change *will* be slow and *it will come through education*. The single viable solution to ISIS, to Islamist radicalism, to Ba'athist political cronyism, to prejudice and inequality of any sort—and even indeed, to poverty—lies in the changing of minds, which can lead to a change of heart. If the current generation of young Muslims is already lost to hatred, prejudice, and a distorted understanding of the Quran—how else can you explain the violent allure of ISIS?—then let the generation after them be educated in the Quran of peace, in standards of ethics, and in the ways of democracy.

Yes, there's a dilemma in all this. How can education be the cure, when Syrian education is itself broken? I cede that fact. I tried in my own small way to aid in the cure of my alma mater and I failed—and then I left. And my own re-education came in the United States and Canada where I learned, not only Western medicine and Western ethics, but also the Quran of peace. Damascus University is just one of hundreds of institutions that suffer so thoroughly from Ba'athism that there can be no cure short of re-gime change.

There's the rub, indeed. The cure to Ba'athism lies in education, whereas the only possible cure of institutions like Damascus University lies in regime change. Please note that a change of regime in no way guarantees a change of mind or of heart. Look at Iraq today and the shape it's in. Removing Saddam Hussein did not cure the Iraqi nation and its institutions of endemic crony-ism. I do look forward to an eventual change of government in Syria. And, when that happens, let the processes begin that will educate new generations in the ways of justice, mercy, and peace.

Again, I digress. So let me step down from my soapbox and return to my narrative.)

Financed by the Palace, AAMAL had instituted a program of training (or re-training) new hires. Had this program been allowed to progress unham-pered by war, I have little doubt that AAMAL today would stand as a progres-sive institutional model for Syria and the Middle East generally. But, in the meantime, we had a waiting list of young patients. They couldn't wait for the re-education to commence, so those of us dedicated to the cause rolled up our sleeves and got to work.

* * *

The children we treated came from poor families, whom we charged a mere token for our services. We gave hearing tests and gave out hearing aids, gave eye exams, and gave out eye glasses. And we gave behavioral therapy to kids with autism. It was a delight to watch the faces of children who, before visiting AAMAL, had experienced the world as garbled noise. Fitted with their first hear-ing aids, they began to tune in to the loving words of their parents—and they could talk and play and laugh with their siblings and friends. Surprisingly, we tested a number of children and found that they wore the wrong aids or didn't need them at all. Their hearing was actually hampered by the devices other physicians had given them. The same with glasses. We delighted in giving the gift of clear sight and, occasionally, in correcting the errors of colleagues.

Among our greatest successes, I would count the cochlear implants some young patients received. Given the cost of this procedure, none of our clients could ever dream of the possibility. But Bashar's rich cousin, Rami Makhlouf, donated money for these implants, and we devised a committee to select the children best served by this surgery. Needless to say, Mr Makhlouf could afford the donation. With a business empire that includes ownership of Syria Tel, Rami's current fortune (estimated at $5 billion) makes him the richest businessman in Syria.

You might ask, how did Rami Makhlouf become so rich? When his uncle, President Hafez al-Assad, decided to take steps that would begin to move Syria from its Soviet-style command economy, he needed to privatize businesses without extending political power to an independent class of businessmen. The solution? He placed much of this newly-privatized wealth in the hands of the Makhloufs, his wife's family. Muhammad Makhlouf (born in 1932) was the family patriarch, financially successful from his work managing state-owned companies and also private businesses. His son Rami Makhlouf (born in 1969) became the young Czar of lucrative private enterprise, primarily Syria Tel along with duty-free concessions at the borders and many other businesses. (In America, you'd call this "keeping it in the family.") How Rami made his money was irrelevant to me back then. All I knew was that Asma made a phone call, Rami wrote a check, and some disabled children were soon able to hear. Not a bad use of tainted money, all in all.

I would also point to our successes in treating childhood autism. I remember one particular child, a pretty three-year-old girl who was virtually catatonic when we began treating her. After many therapy sessions, her face turned from a mask frozen in sadness into an image of joyous, lively engagement. Watching her interact with her parents and brothers and sisters, you'd never guess that she wasn't always a happy, carefree, "normal" child. Left to their own resources, her parents could never have afforded the therapy.

Speaking of parents, before working for AAMAL, I hadn't realized how children's therapy sessions relieved them, too. Specifically, it gave them a welcome if brief respite from the all-consuming, around-the-clock care of their disabled children. Knowing the sacrifices parents make, I was glad to see them have at least a little time to themselves.

Earlier in this chapter, I recounted a newspaper article about England's Princess Diana visitng an English hospital ward and hugging a small, sick child with HIV. I saw similar compassion in Syria's First Lady. Whenever she visited the AAMAL clinic, she was eager to talk to our young patients, to touch them, encourage them, and get them the help they needed. And her membership on the Board was more than nominal. The AAMAL leadership—a triumvirate consisting of the Executive Director, the Board Director, and the Director of Services (the post which I held)—met quadrennially. Our meetings were held at the Tishreen Palace, with the First Lady presiding. (Situated in the Muhajereen district near the New Shaab Palace, the Tishreen is used to host and house visiting foreign dignitaries. In February, 2013, the Free Syrian Army managed to fire two missiles at the Tishreen Palace. The rebels claimed to have caused damage, whereas the government tells a different story. Such is war.) Our meetings were well publicized, leaving no doubt that AAMAL "belonged" to First Lady Asma, and *vice versa*.

I must say that the First Lady did everything in her power to bring publicity to AAMAL. While her husband took visiting heads of state on tours of factories and military bases, the First Lady's "Royal Visits" included the AAMAL clinic. I remember her touring the clinic with Emine Erdogan, First Lady of Turkey and wife of Prime Minister Tayyip Erdogan. With Lara Bashir al-Adem, First Lady of Lebanon and wife of the former Lebanese Prime Minister, Saad Hariri. And with Princess Yasmin Aga Khan, daughter of Rita Hayworth and Syrian-Shiite Prince Aly Khan. These were prime "photo opportunities" for AAMAL and the First Lady alike. But, personally, I did not feel that she was using AAMAL. Rather, she was making her support of disabled children known throughout the Middle East and beyond.

After my second year at AAMAL, I attended a medical conference at The King Fahd Medical City in Riyadh. It was a homecoming of sorts, given my recent residency there. Once again, I was offered a job. And, once again, I was tempted to take the offer.

When I returned to Damascus I told HM, the AAMAL Executive Director, about this renewed job offer. It's as if a conversation that occurred two years prior was reoccurring. Back then, she wooed me with a position at AAMAL. She'd woo me once again, but with a more ambitious offer.

"We need you here," she said, repeating the refrain of our first conversation. But, as she spoke, her words became more thoughtful and deliberate. "There are four million Syrians whose daily functioning is compromised by disability. They need better health care—desperately. What they need is an advocate at the highest level of government—someone who cares about their plight, as I know you do."

"President Assad," she continued, "has created a new post, Secretary General for the Disabled, and he asks that you accept the appointment." Of course, it was the First Lady's doing. A ministerial-level post would raise the profile of the charity she had founded, making more resources available not just to disabled children, but to the disabled generally. She had unleashed her native charm upon her husband, Bashar, who could not say, "No." Nor could I refuse such an offer.

Syria is a nation of ministers: Health, Education, Higher Education, Social Affairs, Labor, Religious Affairs, etc. etc. And now the Disabled would have its Secretary General: me. All the ministries were behind this plan, for the simple reason that the President and First Lady were behind this plan. From each ministry, I would be assigned a liaison officer. It was vital to the workings of government that the ministries kept in close daily contact, coordinating their work.

The year was 2009. I was forty-four years old. I was an idealist, not an ideologue. I had spent my adulthood alternating between the medical clinic and the college classroom—the latter as student and as teacher. I was a trained physician and a medical ethicist. I had spent almost half of the past two decades in North America and the rest in the Middle East. Jordan, Lebanon, Saudi Arabia, Syria. I lived for a time in each, but it was to Syria that I always came back. It was Syria that I called home. And Syria seemed to call to me. In my heart, I believed what the AAMAL Executive Director had said. I *was* needed here. But I was not a Ba'athist. I was a Sufi-inspired Muslim who embraced Western ideals of democracy along with Western technology, medical science, and medical ethics.

And here I was, standing just at the fringe of the Ba'athist power-elite. To stand closer than I was at that moment, I would have had to have been born into the Assad extended family or come up in the ranks of the military. And what I came to realize, during my brief tenure as Secretary General for the Disabled in Syria, was the *powerlessness* of the power-elite when it came to genuine accomplishment.

As a physician, I was taught that "work" meant genuine accomplishment—that something positive actually got done. But, within the world of Ba'athist bureaucracy, I found that all "work" was talk and paper shuffling.

"So, what did you do today?" If you asked the typical bureaucrat that question, he'd puff out his chest and respond, "I met with the Minister of Health, the Associate Minister of Education, and our liaison to the Ministry of Social Affairs!"

"But what did you *accomplish*?" If you asked *that* question, you'd likely be met with a lowered brow and a sullen, suspicious stare.

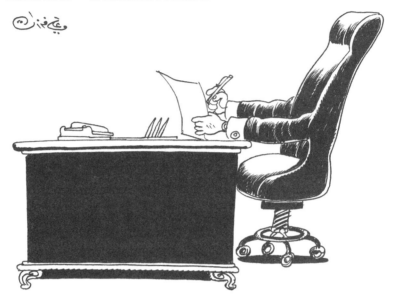

I learned that the typical bureaucrat could not possibly afford his black Mercedes on salary alone. Rather, as long as you kept up with your daily meetings calendar and remained loyal to the First Family, no one noticed (or much cared) what you took home in kickbacks.

Now, the mission of which I took charge was not meant to make anyone rich. Neither was it meant for mere paper-pushing or "busy work." It was intended for *accomplishment*. Still, it remained a government bureaucracy within a larger bureaucratic machine. For this (or any other) mission to behave in any other way than "bureaucratic," it would have had to recreate the Ba'athist organism from which it was born and by which it was nourished and sustained. Let's say that an octopus suddenly grew a new tentacle. How would it differ from the rest? How *could* it differ? It would still be attached to the same octopus, right? And what could it achieve, beyond acting like a tentacle? And even if you called it a "good" tentacle, a "noble" tentacle, a "well-intentioned" tentacle . . . *it's still a tentacle*.

Such was the ministry to which I was appointed. Though well-intentioned, it was remained an appendage of the Ba'athist bureaucracy. So if you were to ask, "What were your greatest accomplishments as Secretary General for the Disabled in Syria?" Here's an answer: "My greatest accomplishments are listed on the following page."

Imagine a blank page.

The plans we drew up for serving the disabled of Syria were as noble and as irrelevant as the Code of Ethics I had drawn up for AAMAL.

We did get a national postage stamp that drew attention to the needs of the disabled, with revenues from sales going to support our mission. The stamp did do some good, but it was mostly symbolic, and the last thing a disabled person needs is a dose of symbolism.

We also managed to install audio aids to help the visually impaired at some of the busier traffic crosswalks in Damascus. In this, we were ahead of most other Arab nations. And yet, several of these audio crosswalk aids were installed backwards. They said "WALK!" when the traffic signal showed "DON'T WALK!" and vice versa. For all I know, people were run over by our good intentions.

I had been beaten, once again. The bureaucratic inertia was too strong to allow for real change.

I was Secretary General for the Disabled in Syria for all of six months before resigning my post and moving back to America—as far from Assad's Syria as I could manage. I was leaving, but I did not wish to see the nation's disabled citizens abandoned and voiceless. So I lobbied actively to be replaced by Hazem Ibrahim, who was named Secretary General for the National Council of Disabilities Services (NCDS). A fellow alumnus of Damascus University, Hazem was the right choice. Although by profession he was a translator, not a physician. Rather, he was himself disabled—paralyzed at age three by a Muslim Brotherhood bullet that had been intended for his father (a Ba'ath party official) but had struck him instead.

It should not be surprising that the NCDS found its best advocates not from among the nation's politicians or health care providers, but from among the disabled themselves. And, since Hazem spent his entire life confined to a wheelchair, he knew firsthand the difficulties some 2 - 4 million Syrians face on a daily basis. He was active in his post until the onset of civil war. But now, sadly, he too has fled the country. And in the course of Syria's civil war, the plight of Syria's disabled has gone from very bad to much, much worse—with no end in sight.

* * *

This chapter began with Asma al-Assad, so I suppose it should end with her. As I've watched the civil war unfold, I've gone back and forth on my opinion of her character. So I surfed the web once more and found an article published November 15, 2012 in VICE News.[20] So far as I could gather, VICE.com is a Canadian-based e-zine that specializes in progressive political watch-dogging. In the article, "Thousands Are Losing Their Thumbs in

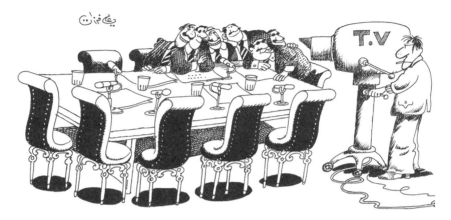

Assad's War While His Wife Pretends to Care About Syria's Disabled," author Milene Larsson interviews Chavia Ali, a Syrian Kurd whom I met once or twice while at AAMAL. Wheelchair-bound by polio, Ali was now chairwoman of the Cultural Forum for People with Special Needs in Syria—a group I hadn't heard of before.

"In 2010," Larsson writes, "Chavia's organization received funding through a trust fronted by Syria's first lady, Asma al-Assad." "*That's convenient,*" I thought to myself. It didn't take long at all for the First Lady to find my replacement. But Chavia Ali's collaborations with the Palace lasted little more than a year. Despite the regime's offer of funding, Ali "didn't accept how they wanted to turn everything into a media show about how great they are and how much they're doing." Ali continues her story:

> When I told them I wanted to use the money to do real work and solve real problems, they stopped paying us. Then, when the revolution began, they started calling me every week because they were in desperate need of arranging public activities that would show they were doing something good, as a way of saying, "Look, we don't have problems in Syria." They begged me, "Please do this project with us. Imagine all the headlines you'll get for disabled people's rights." I told them, "People are dying, and you want me to talk to the press about how caring you are? Do you think I'm crazy?"

While I myself didn't feel used by Asma's "photo ops," I understand that wartime adds a sense of desperation. Before the civil war, it was the First Lady giving publicity to the nation's disabled. With civil war raging, it's the nation's disabled giving publicity to the First Lady.

While it was tough for the disabled before civil war, you can imagine what the violence has brought to the poorest and weakest of God's children. Sadly, Ali's account merely scratches the surface:

> People with disabilities are being left behind when buildings are evacuated. Those who depend on iron lungs, for example, must rely on spare batteries during frequent power outages. Medicine is hard to come by, and soldiers have no regard for whether or not a person is disabled. My friend Adul is almost completely paralyzed and can only move his head. He wanted to participate in the demonstrations in Aleppo, so he went out onto the street in his electric wheelchair. A policeman hit him in the face, and he fell to the ground. When two women came to help him up, they took Adul and the women to prison and locked them up for a month. They don't care whether you're a woman, a child, or in a wheelchair. They'll kill you if you're against them.

I know she's right. Ali stayed to help as long as she could but, once the regime began bombing her home town of Aleppo, she fled for Sweden. It was in Sweden that she gave Larsson this interview.

In so many ways, Chavia Ali's experience mirrored my own at every Syrian institution where I studied or worked. Whereas I had chosen medicine as a means to make a difference, Ali had chosen law. Asked what made her into an activist, she replied:

> I chose to study law at a university in Aleppo that had an elevator, which would enable me to attend lectures and classes. I had such high expectations, but on my first day, when I pressed the elevator button, I realized it was broken. A passerby told me it had been broken for at least ten years. The university staff kept giving me vague excuses [about fixing it], and months passed and nothing happened. Finally, I went to the office of a local politician, a man with enough power to fix my problem in the bat of an eye, and do you know what he told me? He said, "Why do you want to study and have a career in law when you can't even move around?" I became so depressed I stayed in bed for two months, trying to figure out what to do with my life. Finally, I decided to stop focusing on my problem with this elevator and instead work to confront the problems in this society for people with disabilities. If we achieve democracy, we will finally be able to give more power to people with disabilities, like the right to vote. In the old Syria, we never had any of that.

Like Ali, I look forward to seeing the "old Syria," Ba'athist Syria, supplanted by democracy. *That* would be an achievement, and *only* that would lure me back to my homeland.

So much for Chavia. Now for Asma. In March, 2011—just days before the protests broke out—*Vogue* ran a glowing profile of Asma and her family titled, "A Rose in the Desert." A month later, after secret police snipers began picking off peaceful protesters to keep their numbers down and Dara'a had been put under siege, *Vogue* withdrew its article—which was a first for this venerable publication.

Asma had come to Syria, one assumes, to do good work on top of a conservative society, filtering progressive programs and sentiments here and there where she found a crack in the façade, a small space that was not already in the grasp of a vested interest. Syria was a place of tightly locked power arrangements that fiercely resisted change. In a period when Syrians looked to Asia and saw "tigers" like South Korea transform themselves from poverty to world-class prosperity, Syria was standing still. Syria was likely to move forward incrementally, if at all.

Before her marriage, Asma had worked in finance and possessed analytical capabilities. She knew Bashar, knew about Syria, and took a calculated risk. She placed a bet that she could do successful work, make a difference, live her life, and raise her children in a society that, at the time she married, was turning its face to the sun. At the time, her decision did not seem far-fetched.

Bashar's inaugural speech stole lines from JFK. As the new heir apparent, he had famously observed traffic laws on a visit to Aleppo ("He stopped at a red light!" people exclaimed), and insisted on paying for his purchases in the ancient covered market. When he visited an art exhibit by Ali Ferzat and whispered encouragement, the nation's artists and those who yearned for an opening to the West took note. As leader in waiting, Bashar became the nation's unofficial ombudsman. He righted wrongs and fought corruption. And he never missed an opportunity to educate the populace. "Rule of law," Bashar was saying, "is the essence of government, not the exercise of power by a nation's leaders." In his first months as president, Bashar had emptied the country's dungeons and torture chambers. The notorious Mezze prison was slated to become a hospital. Movie theaters were now legal. Private universities were to be authorized some time soon, along with private banks. Private publications were now legal. With Bashar's personal encouragement, Ali Ferzat was licensed to launch *ad-Domari (The Lamplighter)*, credited as the first independent publication since the onset of Ba'ath rule in 1963.

After a decade under Bashar's rule, the country felt much different.

Conspicuous consumption was now allowed. Syria had pulled its troops out of Lebanon—all the way out—and some said, "Syria brought Beirut home with it." The new Damascus was surrounded by fancy restaurants and its highways were clogged with expensive new cars. The First Lady held galas for her charities and international events as if Damascus was Davos in the Levant. Syrians had become more relaxed with foreigners. People could say whatever they wanted, as long as they tiptoed around the Assad family and steered clear of Rami Makhlouf.

Certainly, Syria had problems. Petty crime emerged in a society that, by American standards, had been largely crime-free. Syria's wheatlands had been struck with severe drought from 2006, and families were leaving their farms for the cities—especially nearby cities such as Deir ez-Zor and Dara'a. Bashar's administration addressed the problem, however. And Damascus artists raised money for drought relief. In the first decade of Bashar's rule, it seemed that the old Syria of blood and brutality had been laid to rest. As Bashar's second decade began, *Vogue* came calling. With the encouragement of the New Shaab Palace, the most hopeful Syrians had erected a glittering façade around Bashar and his wife. Could it last?

Dateline: Dara'a. 2011.

On March 6, fifteen boys as young as nine years of age had scrawled anti-government graffiti on a wall and grain silo, a slogan that they had seen on TV from protests in Tunis and Cairo. *"As-Shaab Yoreed eskaat al-nizam!"* The people want to topple the regime! The boys were apprehended by the security services and, as a reward for their artwork, they were disappeared. The parents were told nothing. Rumors of torture were later confirmed when the boys returned—some were missing fingernails.

On March 8, anti-government protests erupted. By March 20 the numbers of protesters had grown from hundreds to thousands and the security forces' violence in suppressing their actions was met by violence in turn.

Ba'athist corruption was the protesters' target, and they took their anger out on the most obvious symbols, including Ba'ath Party headquarters and the local Syria Tel building, owned by Rami Makhlouf. You might say that Dara'a had become a "family matter," and so General Maher al-Assad, the President's younger brother, led the Syrian army in a siege of the city lasting eleven days, from April 25 to May 5.

On Syrian Independence Day, April 17, 2011—just before the Siege of Dara'a—I wrote an email to the First Lady. In my collaborations with the Palace, I had emailed her private secretary before and always received a response. Lady Asma cared for children—I *believe* she cared for children—so

I had written on behalf of the missing boys. I pleaded for these boys, and I pleaded for the protestors who supported these boys. I asked, humbly, that the soldiers not use live ammunition against the protestors. Citing the example of Martin Luther King, Jr, I implored her to protect Syrians who walked the path of nonviolence.

I knew from experience that her voice was heard in the Palace. *Now*, before matters got far worse, was the time for restraint. Asma did not answer my email. Bashar did not make a gallant gesture to defuse the situation. The moment was lost, hundreds died in the siege, and Syria began a steep slide into civil war. All glitter aside, the protestors in Dara'a had not missed the point that the reins of power still lay with the Assad family and that the Ba'ath elite was as strong as ever.

Bashar had made public moves to create a secure, open, liberal state, call it "Syrian democracy." He had brought Syrians with Western credentials into prominent positions in the government. Private banks were created. At least one private university was built. The new cell phone enterprise was created as a private business, rather than a state-owned enterprise. Yet other initiatives were rolled back. Ali Ferzat's *ad-Domari*, for example, only lasted three years before the censors shut it down. It seemed that the reforms that endured were those in which his clan had a business interest. Was Bashar a sincere reformer? Or was he a happy face for the same old Ba'athist machine?

The keystone of the old order was article 8 of the constitution, which gave primacy to the Ba'ath Party. A few years into his rule, Bashar proposed a revision that would allow all parties equal footing. Dates were set for the revision, hopes were raised. When the time came near, however, the proposed revision was always moved forward into the future. As of March, 2011, the revision still had not taken place.

Faced with protest in Dara'a, Bahsar removed his happy face. He called in the troops, just as his father had done years before.

In 2012, Bashar did revise the constitution by public referendum and article 8 was removed. By now, however, blood was flowing in the streets.

Asma al-Assad—our Lady Di—a woman in whom the nation once placed so much hope, did not leave the country in protest. She stepped back to focus on raising her children. She at last had become the Ba'athist wife of the Ba'athist head of state.

Coda:
Where Are We Now?

> The Muslim Ummah [community] is like one body. If the eye is
> in pain, then the whole body is in pain, and if the head is in pain,
> then the whole body is in pain.
>
> —Hadith

On a cloudy morning in April 2015, I found myself sitting in the front passenger seat of a car traveling from Amman, Jordan to the al-Za'atari refugee camp just south of the Syrian border. In point of fact, I was being chauffeured in a clean, late-model Japanese car rented by the Syrian American Medical Society (SAMS).[21] I was heading toward a SAMS-run clinic serving nearly 83,000 thousand refugees crowded together at al-Za'atari. My driver—Mr Abou Maher, who was himself a Syrian refugee—picked me up early that morning at the home of my cousin Sahar and her husband Soufian, with whom I'd be staying for the next eight days while working as a SAMS volunteer. Our ninety-minute drive took us through northern Amman and its outskirts into the Jordan desert. The day being overcast and rainy, we rode with the windows up. Mr Abou Maher told me about his own flight from Syria and the plight of refugees whom I'd be serving. I suppose he was preparing me, as best he could, for what lay ahead. And I listened as best I could, though my eyes concentrated on the desert plain stretching out before me. It was a scene at once strange and familiar, normally dusty-dry but, today, dark, wet, and windy. Drifting in and out of the conversation, I found myself thinking in my own way about the task lying ahead and about the chain of events that was leading me to a Jordanian refugee camp on the Syrian border at the height of civil war.

Having vowed—twice—never to return, I now found myself, if not quite on Syrian soil, then at least back among my people and bearing witness to their increasingly desperate plight.

It seems that the memoirist goes on writing even as the memoir is supposed to have ended. I took 2010 as the terminus of this book and here I am, adding a coda—a literary afterthought—about people and places in 2015. I'm not even writing from the same place. I started in Springfield, Missouri but am finishing up in Milwaukee, Wisconsin. I have returned to teaching and am now associate professor at the Medical College of Wisconsin. As I've heard it said, the only constant is change.

In this coda, I want to account for the people mentioned in previous chapters and to recap my life as well. The five years since I left Syria in 2010 might make for a sequel, though it would be a different sort of memoir than what I've offered here. For it's one thing to write as a Syrian physician living and working in (and leaving) Syria. It's another thing to write as a Syrian-American living and working in the States and watching—though from a great, grievous distance—the Syrian civil war as it has unfolded. Much has happened over the past five years, and the path I've taken has been circuitous, indeed.

My first stop was St Vincent's Hospital in Billings, Montana. Given my résumé and expertise in pediatric neurology, it was not hard to find work, though I had forgotten just how cold the winters could get in the American Northwest. I began at St Vincent's in fall 2010. At the time, Bashar al-Assad's hold on Syria seemed iron-tight and I saw no chance for change.

But change surprised us all, as the "Arab Spring" made its way steadily across North Africa and into the Middle East. By January 2011, civilian protests were erupting in Syria, leading to government crackdowns. Even as I was settling into my job at St Vincent's, Syrian friends and family began phoning and posting on Facebook, frantically. And then came March 8 and the outrage at Da'ara, where teenaged boys were arrested, imprisoned, and tortured, their "crime" being anti-government graffiti. The protests spread and the crackdowns intensified.

Throughout these early months, my emotions were mixed and uncertain. Of course I longed for freedom for my people, but I had seen Ba'athist oppression firsthand and feared for the safety of protestors, holding out little hope for their success. Others in my situation might have felt guilty for having bailed out before the storm hit home. But I had already tried in my own small way to affect change, and I had failed. So, no, I felt no personal guilt for having left the bloodshed behind.

Still, as March gave way to April and popular protests reached the streets of Damascus, I felt rumblings of an inner urgency, as if I should *do* something, though what that *something* was I did not yet know. Billings is about as far away from Damascus as one can get. April gave way to May and the city of Homs fell under siege, followed by Tafas and Rastan and Talbiseh. If there were *any* role that I could play, I knew it would be educative and humanitarian, not activist or political.

While I could not influence events in Syria, I could at least interpret them for fellow Americans. But how? By what means? Having witnessed the failures of Syrian education and health care and having been privy to Ba'athist cronyism, I thought of writing. I could tell my stories, and I knew that my stories left an impression, but I had no clue as to how to shape and organize and write them down.

June came and it was Aleppo that erupted. Wildfires of civil dissent were spreading across Syria and here I was, a passive spectator. July came and went, as did August and September, each with its sieges and massacres. By September, soldiers once loyal to Assad were defecting *en masse* to form the Free Syrian Army (FSA), which vowed regime change by force. Given my deepening commitments to Sufism and the Quran of peace, I grieved over their efforts to outgun Assad. The only form of protest that I could support in conscience remained nonviolent, in the manner of Gandhi and King. But what began as peaceful civilian protests had grown into full-blown civil war, and let there be no doubt as to which side I was on. The FSA had at last wiped the smirk off the face of Ba'athism. As the FSA grew in numbers and in the boldness of its attacks, it seemed that regime change was, for once, a real possibility.

As 2011 came to an end, I came to recognize my own greatest frustration. It wasn't that I was a spectator as opposed to participant. It's that I was failing *even in that role*. I did not, in fact, have a clear window into events unfolding halfway across the globe.

Here's the hardest part of living in the States over these past five years. While all of Syria reeled from terrorism and war, I could never get enough news—enough *real* news, unbiased and reliable. I came to think of American television—of whatever ilk, progressive or conservative, network or cable—as a tease. TV anchors declared the latest massacre as a lead story of the day, whereas the actual newscast skimmed the surface. An image or two, a reporter's sound-bite, the TV anchor's expression of sympathy or shock or dismay, and then on to the commercials. (If it were not for the rise of ISIS, I suspect that Syria would have dropped from American TV news. It grieves me to write this, but the need for "fresh content" dictates American viewing tastes. The names of Syrian towns—most unknown by most Americans—and the numbers of civilian casualties might change, but the news seemed unchanging from day to day: "Today's siege in . . . today's massacre in . . . today's bombing in . . ." Just fill in the blanks and there's your news *du jour*. To the TV viewer, the very monotony of war makes it mind-numbing. There is little "fresh content" when it comes to war-reporting.)

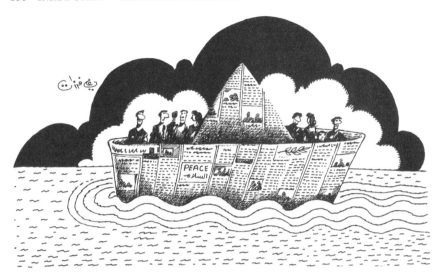

American newspapers offered more depth in reporting but still left me hungering. I found myself surfing English and Arab websites and intensifying my correspondence with friends, family, and former colleagues. But even among friends and family, Assad still had his followers. This surprised me—shocked me, in fact. Only my closest relations could be relied upon to hazard the full, unvarnished truth. Otherwise, whatever the source, the news out of Syria was slanted or censored and generally woeful.

In the meantime, I had my own life to live. By early 2012 I had moved from St Vincent's Hospital in Billings to Mercy Hospital in Springfield. Comfortable. That's how I'd describe the life I was building for myself and my little family. The Ozarks climate was temperate and everything about my job was predictable. I began leading Friday prayers for Muslim inmates in the county jail. I was respected in the community. But while the climate of my personal world was temperate and comfortable, all Syria was in flames.

Firestorms burn themselves out . . . in time, when there's nothing left to burn. In 2012, the regime was on the defensive and, by all appearances, losing. Neighborhood after neighborhood fell to the rebels and army defections continued. A majority of Syrians stood against the regime and it seemed a mere matter of time before the House of Assad would fall. And the regime would have to answer for its crimes against humanity, despite Ba'athist attempts to conceal its acts of terror against civilians.

Had Syrians been left to their own resources, the firestorm would indeed have burned out. Of this, I am convinced. But Syria's neighbors poured fuel on the fire. What began as popular protests and had morphed into civil war was now a proxy war among regional powers and the religious sects that they purport to represent. I cannot begin to describe the various alliances and complicities that have drawn Sunni, Shiite, Alawite, Kurdish, Turkish, Iraqi, Saudi, Qatari, Iranian, Jordanian, and Lebanese interests into the Syrian conflict. Resupplied and propped up by Shiite Iran and the Lebanese Hezbollah, the regime managed to dig itself in and hold onto a strategic portion—say a third, more or less—of the land and population. Neither the rebels nor the regime had the firepower for a knock-out blow, so the conflict ground down to a war of attrition. For my own part, throughout the year 2012, I spent my days in the US practicing pediatric medicine, studying medical ethics, and speaking (to whomever would listen) of the Quran of peace.

It was early in 2013 that Bashar al-Assad, desperate to break the stalemate, used chemical weapons against his own people. The decision was bone-chilling in its logic. Simply put, it proved easier to wipe out whole neighborhoods than to root out the rebels perched on rooftops and hidden in alley ways. The worst instance occurred in the Ghouta suburb of Damascus in August, when as many as 1,700 men, women, and children were sarin-gassed. I was shocked by the initial reporting. But, as the details leaked out, I found myself thrown into a meditation.

The Ghouta is downhill from the Presidential compound. It can be glimpsed from that big bay window that I once looked out of, while drinking coffee with the President. And now I pictured him sitting quiet and pensive, sipping on that same exquisite Arabian coffee served in a dainty china cup emblazoned with the Presidential Seal of Syria. I imagined him breathing in the aroma from that cup as sarin gas wafted over the neighborhood nearby. As steam rose from his cup, I imagined smoke rising, visible from his bay window. And soon corpses—as many as 1,700—of Ghouta's men, women, and children would be frozen in place where the gas had surprised them, suffocating them. Their bodies would be gathered up and placed in an arena-sized room in row after row all neat and efficient, *abattoir*-like, each swathed in white cloth, each stiff and cold.

Some of the fiercest ironies that I've confronted in writing this memoir pertain to my perceptions of the man, Bashar al-Assad, himself. I saw him as an awkward, seemingly lost teenager. While studying medicine, I knew him as an unpretentious and personable fellow student. And, when I returned to Syria to teach, I did so through his patronage—and found him pleasant and affable. Nothing that I saw in him during any of our meetings seemed extraordinary. How, then, does one account for this turn to atrocity? What lured him down this terrifying path? Was it an inferiority complex (reflected,

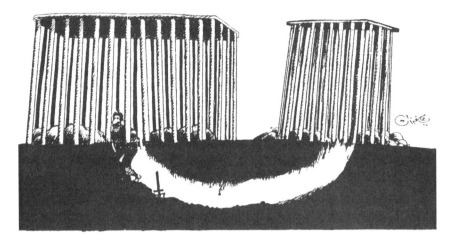

perhaps, in his speech impediment) that led him to the ultimate over-compensation—the decimation of his own people? Was it fear—fear, perhaps, of his own people, or of the ghost (that is, the legacy) of his tyrant-father—that led him to such spectacular feats of violence? Or was it guilt, of the sort that comes from being born into a murderous family? Such guilt might lead one to murder in turn, ensuring one's own inevitable punishment.

It was around the time of this last atrocity that a friend of mine introduced me to WD Blackmon. I remember having lunch with Professor Blackmon, who listened intently to the stories of my childhood and early dealings with Assad.

"You ought to write a book," WD said. "Americans need to hear your story." I explained that I had started writing in Montana, but it was going very slowly. WD kept encouraging me: "Americans may not understand the Middle East or Syria or Assad in the abstract, but they'll understand and respond to personal experience such as yours."

And then the barrel bombs started falling—by the tens and, soon, by the hundreds—on defenseless civilian populations. By spring 2014, WD and I were both feeling the urgency of answering the state sanctioned violence—with words. WD agreed to help. And we worked together for more than a year, producing a chapter every other month or so while war continued to rage.

We worked through Syria's sham "free elections," through Israel's latest pounding of Gaza, through the transformation of the deadly al-Nusra Front into the even deadlier ISIS. But we kept our focus on the past, out of a conviction that past experience could help explain the present.

Such was the path that led to this memoir. But even as I wrote, I was preparing for a further life-change. A move from Springfield, Missouri, to Milwaukee, Wisconsin. It was there in February 2015 that I became reacquainted with SAMS—the Syrian American Medical Society that sponsored my work at al-Za'atari.

I had been involved with SAMS when it was first established in 1999 and I was in the States teaching at Case Western. But, returning to Syria in 2002, I drifted away from the group. Truth to tell, I felt that some members were using SAMS to curry favor with the regime. From the near-distance of my own minor government post, I'd hear of the fanfare surrounding their arrival in Damascus, where they'd be escorted to the New Shaab Palace and wait their turn for a photo-op handshake with Bashar.

I believe that organizations, like individuals, can experience a "purification of the heart." And I believe that the current civil war has served to reinvigorate SAMS and its medical-humanitarian mission in Syria, separate from any political kowtowing. So in early 2015—when I was myself, once again, a Syrian expatriate teaching in the States—I was ready to turn my attention back to SAMS.

For the past four years, Dr Zaher Sahloul—a pulmonary specialist and graduate of Damascus University Medical School—has served as SAMS President. He and I attended med school together, so I wrote him an email: "What," I asked, "was being done to address the psychological and psychosocial wounds of Assad's victims, the children especially?"

His response was quick, pleasant, and hopeful. He told me that SAMS was building a US-based team of psychiatrists and psychologists and was actively supporting specialists in Jordan and Lebanon. He put me in contact with Dr Khalid Hamzeh, a forensic psychologist who headed a Syrian-American medical team operating in Jordan. I became a member of his team.

In early February, a Milwaukee chapter of SAMS was receiving its charter and I had been invited to the dinner gala. My old schoolmate Zaher, President of SAMS, led the ceremony. We exchanged pleasantries (not having seen each other since med school), but our conversation soon turned serious.

"I know you're wanting to treat the psychological scars of our people," he said, making a slow wind-up to his next pitch: "in the meantime, we don't have a child neurologist working in any of the SAMS clinics—not in Jordan or Lebanon or Turkey. We need you."

"I will come," I said.

"Good, my friend, good. When?"

"In April, when I have some time off from teaching. I will go to Jordan then."

"Good, my friend, good." Sealing my promise with a handshake, he went off to mingle with other guests. And I spent the rest of the evening mentally planning my trip.

I wanted to visit al-Za'atari—the largest refugee camp in the Middle East (and, arguably, in the world), serving some 83,000 "persons of concern," according to the United Nations High Commissioner for Refugees.[22] I've read that, by sheer numbers, al-Za'atari might claim to be the fifth largest "city" in Jordan today.[23] But of course it's not a "city" legally and it lacks the resources that one would expect of the fifth largest *anything* in a nation like Jordan. It's simply a "camp," a "permanent settlement camp," UN-sponsored and hosted by the Hashemite Kingdom. I'd be spending my days working at al-Za'atari, but I'd have precious evenings to spend with cousin Sahar and her family. I wouldn't be going home to Damascus, but I'd be visiting relatives and it would be a homecoming of sorts.

On the morning after my arrival in Amman, I woke up at 4:00 AM to the call for prayers and began preparing for the ride to al-Za'atari. And, with that as my segue, I return to the passenger seat of the SAMS rental car, the subject with which this coda began.

By mid-morning, we arrived at al-Za'atari. It was fence-enclosed but a bearded man, rail-thin and riding a bike, soon cycled up to the locked entrance gate. Following a brief interrogation, he welcomed us in. His appearance made an impression on me and I learned later that he had been one of the first to stand against the government in Dara'a. In fact, most of the refugees at al-Za'atari came from the Dara'a region.

I cannot explain to readers the complexity of my response, almost half-joyous and more than half-grievous. Like my emotions, the camp itself was a jumble of contradictions, both squalid and bustling. It's hard to call the refugees inside "lucky" and yet, compared to their compatriots outside, they were lucky to have what little they had. And they were determined to have a life if not quite make a living. It was raining on that first day, which made mud of the camp's typically sun-hardened fields—fields that had been improvised into shanty-streets lined with tents and small, pre-fabricated cubicles placed on pallets, each large enough to house two people, though a half-dozen might live or work together in one of these corrugated tin-and-plywood "boxes."

Make-shift and make-do. That's how I'd describe just about everything at al-Za'atari, though the effect was not entirely bad. One could see signs of ingenuity and sheer human resourcefulness mixed in with the worry, grief, anger, fear, despair, and boredom of camp life. The narrow mud-turned "roads" separating the tent-row "streets" could barely accommodate a car, but as we drove gingerly by, the camp's children came running out to chase us, waving at us. Our car had become their entertainment. So had the mud puddles. What else was there for these children to do?

"And now we're traversing the *Champs Elysees*," declared my driver Abou Maher, with a pretty good imitation of a French accent. The nickname was both ironic and apt. Just as the most famous street in Paris holds that city's finest shops, so this street had grown into the camp's shopping district—a bazar where almost anything could be bought and where everything sold was contraband. Of course the prices were inflated. But the people were living as best they could, and who could blame them for doing so?

Make-shift. That's how I'd describe the SAMS clinic facilities when we had at last arrived. There was a line of people standing before each of the clinic's cubicles. It had been raining steadily, so there they stood, rain-soaked and ankle-deep in mud, waiting their turn. Later, I was told that they had begun lining up around 4:30 AM, just as I was finishing my morning prayers in Amman. And some who had arrived six hours ago were apparently still standing in line, waiting their turn.

There was much to do so the introductions were brief. Dr Khaled Ibrahim, an ear, nose, and throat specialist, was the clinic's medical director. His team that day included a neurosurgeon, two pediatricians, an OB/GYN specialist, a urologist, and two dentists. And now he could add a child neurologist—me—to that list. As I took my station in one of the pre-fab cubicles, I was told to expect as many as twenty patients that day. My examination room held a small pressed-wood laminated table for instruments, a long, narrow metal fold-up table for patients, and a stackable white plastic lawn chair for me. (If I didn't know better, I'd swear these furnishings had come from my local Walmart back home. Even the sheets and blankets on the metal table looked like they came from Walmart. Then again, one doesn't usually use metal hobbyist tables and store-bought lawn chairs in medical exam rooms.)

Make-do: that's what you learn when put in a pre-fab "box" with a line of sick, rain-soaked children queued outside. In the States, it takes me an hour on average to see one child. So I imagined myself in an emergency-room setting and resolved to help as many as I could as much as I could as quickly as I could. What else was there for me to do?

A veiled woman on the younger side of middle age assisted me. She was introduced to me as Faten. Her voice was strong when calling in each patient, and I must admit that her air of confidence boosted my own. "Call in Tarek Majeed, nurse Faten," I remember saying early on in our team work.

"Nurse, doctor?" was her reply: "I am not a nurse. I have a degree in history." Make-do, indeed. My admiration for her increased.

Around noontime, while I was taking a breather between patients, Dr Ibrahim came over to my cubicle.

"Dr Bakdash . . . Tarif." the medical director began, "you probably don't remember, but you were my teacher."

"Really?" I said, genuinely surprised. "When?"

"When you taught bioethics at Damascus University," he replied. "I took your class." Dr Khaled and I shared a few quick reminiscences and then went back to work.

Later that day, two other team members—Dr Harriri and a person I'll call Dr Adel—came over to my cubicle. "Do you remember us?" they asked in tandem: "We were your students at Damascus University."

Back in Wisconsin, I wasn't surprised to meet Dr Sahloul, an old classmate. The fact that Dr Sahloul reintroduced me to SAMS didn't surprise me, either. But that I would find myself joined at a SAMS clinic by three former students—one of whom was directing the clinic I was working at—lay beyond imagination. Never in my wildest dreams did I expect to travel from a university hospital in the American Midwest to a refugee camp in Jordan to find myself serving side-by-side with students whom I had taught bioethics in Damascus, Syria. Though they, too, had fled the Ba'athist regime, still they were using their talents in behalf of their countrymen. And if these three were anything like the hundreds that I had taught in that sweaty, cavernous auditorium, then those hundreds will have helped thousands—many thousands, perhaps—in a manner worthy of Islam.

These three (and many more, I was willing to hope) were actively *living* the Quran of peace. Anyone who has read this memoir will know that I left Damascus University in frustration, doubting that I had made even in the slightest dent in the Ba'athist health care machinery. But here before me stood living proof that my homeland could produce a generation of competent, dedicated, ethical physicians—and not because of the Ba'athist system but in spite of it. I don't know when I've ever felt prouder, or when I've felt more humbled.

Yet it's not my old classmate or former students or favorite cousins that left the deepest impression. It's the children with their parents who stood that first day out in the rain waiting their turn. The children were so sweet to me, yet you could see the sadness in their eyes. And the parents smiled, though their faces showed fear and anxiety—and weariness—intermingled with hope. What else did they have, if not hope?

I was able to help some. Others, I couldn't. A mother brought in two of her children, both with scoliosis so severe that they might soon die without surgery. I had to look the mother in the eye and say, "I am sorry, there's not much I can do."

"But we were hoping that you are from the United States and can help us," she replied. Her hope was naïve and I hated to take it from her. After all, what else did she have?

The fact is that her children *could* be saved, if adequate hospital facilities—and money—were available. And I wouldn't have had to fly them back with me to Wisconsin. We could have driven to Amman. But who would pay? Time and again I found myself saying, "I am sorry, there's not much I can do," knowing full well that an EEG or MRI would have cost only one hundred US dollars in a Jordanian hospital. I could have helped—somewhat, at least. I could have ordered tests to arrive at a diagnosis, if not a cure. But the parents of the children who saw me had no money.

Toward the end of that first day, the sun had at last come out and I stepped outside to feel its rays and breathe in the fresh air. As I stood outside the clinic, a young woman approached me and asked, "Can you help me, doctor?"

"I'm sorry," I said, "but I see only children."

"I have multiple sclerosis," she replied.

I could not say no. "I will see you tomorrow," I said.

Before leaving al-Za'atari that first day, Abou Maher took me for a more leisurely ride around camp. As the rain water receded, I noticed that some of what seemed to be mud puddles were in fact open sewage ditches cut into the side of roadways. These converged into larger rivulets that carried the sewage away from the overcrowded camp's center, though whereto I had no idea.

"The camp's had no electricity for the past few months," Abou Maher declared as we drove.

"Why not?" I asked, dumbfounded.

He shrugged at first, but soon launched into an explanation: "The Jordanian government says it doesn't have the money, so they stopped supplying it. The SAMS facilities run on their own generators."

He said more: "Remember, the camp may be UN-sponsored, but al-Za'atari is on Jordanian soil. Whatever comes into the camp comes with permission of the government and passes through government checkpoints."

"I see," was my own lame response. I was still contemplating the prospects of families crowded together in a pre-fab "box" with no air conditioning in one hundred degree plus daily summertime temperatures.

"There are water deliveries," Abou Maher added, "once a week."

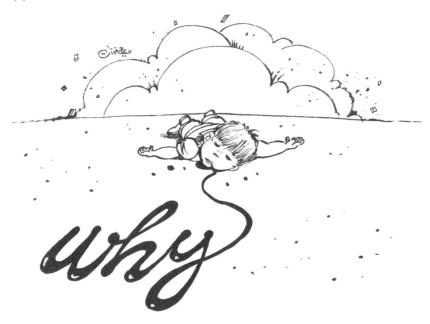

"*No wonder the children welcomed the rain,*" I thought to myself.

When I arrived back at Sahar's house that evening, I told my female cousins what I had seen but held back much of what I had heard. It was too gruesome. Rape, apparently, was a war zone weapon that Assad's soldiers used in "liberating" rebel-held villages. One might have hoped that atrocities like rape proved exceptions to the rule of warfare, but the camp's hundreds upon hundreds of rape victims could not be dismissed as isolated, rogue incidents. Soldiers not only raped but mutilated their victims, sometimes severing spinal cords. I was told of one rape victim who had been left paralyzed. Though she had been "saved" and brought to camp, she had lost the will to live. She refused to eat and died.

I did tell my cousins about the young woman with MS. The SAMS clinic had a supply of only the most basic medicines. The camp had nothing for multiple sclerosis—not even methylprednisolone, a corticosteroid that could at least have relieved her symptoms. Overcome with sympathy, cousin Areej donated the money to buy medication.

I don't want to give false impressions about the camp's resources or lack thereof. The SAMS clinic received a modest supply of pharmaceuticals, which were used efficiently for the greater good of the greatest number of people. And while the available lab tests were limited, I always got results on the same day. "*Pretty impressive for a camp,*" I thought to myself. Surgeries, however, were a different story. At the SAMS clinic, we could do only the most minor, outpatient procedures. Emergency surgeries had to be done outside the camp.

Keep in mind that Syria's own domestic pharmaceutical industries have been virtually wiped out by civil war. A proud nation that once supplied ninety percent of its pharmaceuticals was now lacking in the most basic of surgical supplies, including blood bags, surgical sets, sterilization equipment, operating tables, even IV fluids. People injured across the border in Syria could expect little help at home, so the more dire effects of war spilled over into Jordan. I came to al-Za'atari expecting to treat traumatized children, not battle-wounded soldiers.

Several days into my assignment, the head of one of the UNHCR medical teams—he was an Irishman, Brandon by name—asked us to come over to their field hospital and help evaluate a young Syrian rebel who had been shot in the chest and paralyzed waist-down. It turns out that our clinic's neuro-surgeon, Dr Ayman, had diabetes and was monitoring himself daily. Stress (both physical and emotional) can cause a rise in blood sugar level. And while 250 is dangerously high, my colleague had a glucose reading of 460—which would have sent him to an emergency room if he were in the States, due to the threat of ketoacidosis or diabetic coma. Dr Ayman should have stayed and rested, since his fatigue was both cause and symptom of elevated blood sugar. Instead, he took a shot of insulin and rushed off with us to the field hospital. (I could have tried to dissuade him, but I knew he wouldn't listen. His dedication was too strong.)

When we arrived at the young Syrian's bedside, he was smiling and hope-ful for himself, though he had lost contact with his family and worried for their sake. While my colleagues examined him, I was asked to use my neu-rologist's skills on the young man lying next to him. He had been hit in the head by shrapnel and had lost all ability to communicate. His eyes were open and he followed me with his eyes as I examined him, but he said nothing. I spoke to him but, beyond following me with his eyes, he remained unre-sponsive. Though he was otherwise very much alive, the trauma to his brain had sentenced him to a living death. Once again I found myself saying, "I am sorry, there's not much I can do."

By the third day, I had grown close to my team members and we had sup-per together. The clinic's facilities manager, Abou Khaled, had asked his wife to cook, and the meal she made for us was magnificent in its way—not for its cost or variety, but for the fact that she made-do and fed so many with such modest resources. (Since returning to the States, I learned that Abou Khaled had ran afoul of the Jordanian authorities. Apparently he defended the rights of patients. His reward was to be picked up with his family, packed in a car, and carried back across the border to Syria.)

While sharing that meal, I came to realize what it was that impressed me most about the SAMS clinic at al-Za'atari. It was the genuine team unity, the total commitment of team members, the mutual respect afforded to all, and the lack of hierarchy. This is what I had longed for, and failed to achieve, at AAMAL. Some of the physicians sitting around that dinner table had invitations to live and work in Europe. "Surely you were tempted," I asked someone sheepishly, thinking back to the many offers that I've had, and have accepted, over the years.

"No," replied my Syrian colleague matter-of-factly: "I will never leave my people alone in this camp." There is a joy, he said, in serving the poorest of his countrymen, especially the victims of Assad's regime: "And there is no price equal to joy." So ended that topic of conversation.

Over my last few days at al-Za'atari, parents of the children I had seen kept coming up to thank me for my help. In many cases, I had helped very little if at all. But I suppose that simply being there and caring and strengthening another's hope is reason enough to be thanked. "You're welcome," I'd reply, "and may God bring peace to your heart and health to your child."

Having finished my eight days' service, I promised to return and look forward to keeping that promise. After all, what else is there for a Syrian-American physician to do? *There*, in a camp like al-Za'atari, is the place of need. The people there are in need. And the path of service leads one *there*. In the meantime, I do my daily rounds at the Children's Hospital of Wisconsin and speak to whomever will listen about the plight of Syrians and the Quran of Peace.

Just recently, I was asked to give the Grand Rounds at the Children's Hospital of Wisconsin and the Medical College of Wisconsin. For readers unfamiliar with med school tradition, I should explain that the Grand Rounds are an age-old practice in teaching- and research-hospitals, where a physician is selected to present a difficult case to fellow faculty, residents, and students. For my subject, I choose to speak not of an individual patient but of an entire population at-risk. My title ran, "Helping Syria's Kids: Whose Responsibility Is It?" I was pleased (and surprised) by the size of the audience and gratified by the emails I received afterward, asking how to help. But I found the question-and-answer period most poignant. One colleague asked, "How can you explain the fact that Bashar Assad, himself a physician, could kill so many innocent people?" If the question weren't so somber, I might have thrown out something semi-witty, like "well, I could write a book on *that* topic—in fact,

I *did* write a book!" But that was not the time for levity. What came to mind was a cliché, no less true for being well-worn: "Power corrupts," I said, "and absolute power corrupts absolutely."

***

So much for my own life to-date.

The Syrian civil war is ongoing and Bashar al-Assad remains in power, with First Lady Asma by his side. I suppose they spend most of their days hunkered down in the New Shaab Palace. But of other people mentioned in this memoir, the reader might like to know who is still alive and who is living where. I think there's some closure—for me, at least—in asking, "Where are *they* now?"

My mentor at Henry Ford Hospital, Dr Jeffrey M. DeVries, is still practicing. My mentor at the Baylor College of Medicine, Dr Marvin Fishman, has recently retired after a long career of service. (In 1979, Dr Fishman founded the Baylor section of Neurology and Developmental Neuroscience. He will be remembered for leading this program into national prominence.)

My American-educated uncle, Dr Bashar Bakdash, is still hard at work teaching at the University of Minnesota Medical School. And you'll remember my second American-educated uncle, Dr Hisham Bakdash, who returned to Syria many years ago to teach at the Damascus University Medical School. Since the outbreak of civil war he, too, has come back to America. Retired from medicine, uncle Hisham lives in Ohio with his American-born wife.

I've already mentioned that Chavia Ali—my "replacement" as First Lady Asma's disability poster child—has left Syria for Sweden. You'll also remember my brother-in-law Hassan Sahtout, a pediatric surgeon who made his perilous escape by sea. He, too, lives in Sweden with his family. I should add that HM—the AAMAL Executive Director who hired me and was instrumental in my appointment as Secretary General for the Disabled—left Syria for Yemen. But, given the political shocks Yemenis have met in recent months, she found her first place of refuge turned into a fresh battle zone. She has since moved to Saudi Arabia, which brings pleasure to my heart.

I do not know what happened to Messrs Dadoush and Zaeem, my teachers at Al-Thaqafi. I pray they're alive still and have avoided tragedy. Of my childhood friends, I might mention Nidal Kurdi (with whom I played Atari while Iraqi tanks rolled through Iran). He went on to study medicine, becoming a neurologist. And he, too, has immigrated to the United States.

While many have left the Middle East, I have many friends and family members who remain. My aunt Hiyam still lives in Amman, Jordan. So do my cousins Areej and Reem and Sahar and Samar. And though Samar's handsome son Omar (he who murmured "Mar . . . mar . . . marmalade" as a child) worked for a time in the Saudi Kingdom, he now has come back to Jordan, where he works as an engineer. The rest of my family is still in Syria hoping to see peace one day soon.

And now for the two men who figured in my mother's tragedy. Nawal's Beirut boss—the rich and lazy-eyed Nizar Azem—died of renal failure, despite a kidney donation from his son Hassan. On the other hand, his associate Rafiq al-Nafsteh is still very much alive and immersed in Palestinian affairs. In 2012, he was serving as head of the Palestinian Authority's anti-corruption commission. (Now *that's* an irony, given the path that Nafsteh took to power.)

Ali Ferzat lives in exile in Kuwait where he has continued his career as a political cartoonist.

For each and every one, I pray for God's mercy.

And I pray for the health care workers and volunteers and for the refugees and victims and for those who resist terror and oppression, both in Syria and throughout the Middle East and the world. I pray that peace may come in our lifetime. And I pray that radical Muslims will lay down their weapons and unite in walking the path of peace that God has shown us all and recorded in His book, the Quran of peace. For, in the end,

> . . . all that dwells upon the earth shall perish. Except the face of thy Lord, majestic and splendid.
>
> —Quran 55:26

In Closing

I love Syria, an ancient country, and hope that it can emerge from the chaos that now reigns and become a society that spreads its blessings to all citizens. As you've seen, however, in my experience Syria was a place of perpetual conflict, a Ba'athism with rigid Soviet-style attitudes and procedures that led to inefficient state-owned industries, an entrenched bureaucracy, a privileged elite, and a suffocating paranoia.

When I came to the United States, I found a society that is not perfect but allowed me to experience a freedom of thought, speech, and movement that I had never known before. It provided me opportunities to refine my skills as a physician and as a teacher. It facilitated my emergence as an ethicist and, because of freedom of religion, encouraged a spiritual journey that led me to the Quran of peace and mercy.

I have written about Syria. This book is my *jihad* on behalf of the Quran of the heart. Because I wrote this book, I can't return to Syria as long as Ba'athism holds sway. But I've found a new country where my personal and professional development is moving forward. Given the fate of so many Syrians, I'm deeply grateful.

—Tarif Bakdash, MD
Milwaukee, 2016

Resources

Notes

1. I am following the web-based text of Jonathan Fairbanks and Clyde Edwin Tuck's *Past and Present of Greene County, Missouri* (1915). Http://thelibrary.org/lochist/history/paspres/.
2. *Heart of Islam: Enduring Values for Humanity* (New York: HarperCollins, 2004).
3. See, for example, my book chapter (co-authored with Abdallah S. Daar and Ahmed B. Khitamy), "Islamic Bioethics" in *The Cambridge Textbook of Bioethics*, ed. Peter M. Singer and A. M. Viens (Cambridge, UK: Cambridge University Press, 2008), pp. 408-15. I would also point to my Arabic-language articles in popular magazines and in *Tabebak*, a widely-read Syrian medical journal. My 2006 *Tabebak* article, "What is Bioethics?" is, arguably, the seminal discussion of Western-based biomedical ethics in Syria.
4. *Islamic Biomedical Ethics: Principles and Application* (New York: Oxford UP, 2009), p. 21.
5. Sachedina, *Islamic Biomedical Ethics*, p. 93.
6. *No Victor, No Vanquished: The Yom Kippur War* (New York: Presidio, 1978).
7. *History of Syria: 1900-2012* (Cambridge, MA: Charles River Editors, 2012), ebook.
8. Clement, *History of Syria*.
9. *Syria: The Fall of the House of Assad* (New Haven: Yale University Press, 2012), Kindle ebook.
10. *Israel's Lebanon War* (New York: Simon and Schuster, 1984), p. 284.
11. *Dreams and Shadows: The Future of the Middle East* (New York: Penguin, 2008), pp. 243-44.
12. Ted Regencia, "My Classmate is a War Criminal," *Aljazeera*, August 6, 2012. http://www.aljazeera.com/indepth/features/2012/08/201281141339576130.html. I have kept in touch with Dr Sahloul and have worked with him through the Syrian American Medical Association, a charitable relief organization of which is he currently

president. All three are now Chicagoans: Drs. Sahloul and Alzein practice medicine, while Basatneh (who did not complete his medical studies) works in business.

13. See "The Founders of al-Mouwasat Hospital," http://www.syrianhistory.com/en/photos/692?search=Hospital.

14. See "ECFMG: Educational Mission for Foreign Medical Graduates." www.ecfmg.org.

15. *All Men Are Brothers: Autobiographical Reflections* (New York: Columbia University, 1958).

16. *The Essential Gandhi: An Anthology* (New York: Random House, 1962).

17. *The Papers of Martin Luther King, Jr.* (Berkeley: University of California Press, 1992).

18. See "Faculty of Medicine at Damascus University," *Wikipedia.* http://en.wikipedia.org/wiki/Faculty_of_Medicine_of_Damascus_University.

19. See William Winslade, Mark Siegler, and Albert Jonsen's *Clinical Ethics: A Practical Approach to Ethical Decisions in Clinical Medicine* (New York: McGraw-Hill, 2002).

20. See Milene Larson, "Thousands Are Losing Their Thumbs in Assad's War While His Wife Pretends to Care about Syria's Disabled," VICE.*com.* http://www.vice.com/read/thousands-are-losing-their-limbs-in-assads-war-0000365-v19n11.

21. As the SAMS website declares, "Our vision is to be a leading humanitarian organization, harnessing the talents of Syrian-American health care professionals, and channeling them toward medical relief for the people of Syria and the United States. See "Mission and Vision," SAMS Foundation. www.sams-usa.net/foundation/index.php/who-we-are/mission-vision.

22. See UNHCR, "Zaatari Refugee Camp," *Syria Regional Refugee Response.* http://data.unhcr.org/syrianrefugees/settlement.php?id=176&region=77&country=107. The UNHCR has gathered statistics on the camp's residents by age, of whom 54%—some 42,000—are aged seventeen and under. Needless to say, the UNHCR lacks data for the many tens of thousands of displaced Syrians in regions surrounding al-Za'atari, who have even less than the scant resources afforded those in camp.

23. See the April 22 1983 web-archived article, "Syria's refugees: birth and life in Zaatari camp." www.theguardian.com/global-development/gallery/2013/apr/22/syria-refugees-zaatari-in-pictures.

Bibliography

Armstrong, Karen. *Islam. A Short History.* New York: Random House, 2000.

Arberry, Arthur, trans. *The Koran Interpreted.* New York: Macmillan, 1955.

Bell, Gertrude. *The Desert and the Sown.* London: Virago Press, 1985.

Browning, Iain. *Palmyra.* Park Ridge: Noyes Press, 1979.

Burckhardt, John Lewis. *Travels in Syria and the Holy Land.* London: John Murray, 1822.

Burns, Ross. *Monuments of Syria: An Historical Guide.* New York: NYU Press, 1992.

Cleveland, William L. *A History of the Modern Middle East.* Boulder: Westview Press, 2000.

Davis, Scott C. *The Road From Damascus.* Seattle: Cune Press, 2003.

Farzat, Ali. *A Pen of Damascus Steel.* Seattle: Cune Press, 2005.

Haeri, Shakyh Fadhlalla. *The Elements of Sufism.* New York: Barnes and Noble, 1999.

Hitti, Philip. *History of the Arabs.* London: Macmillan, 1970.

Hopkins, Clark. *The Discovery of Dura-Europos.* Yale: Yale University Press, 1979.

Kamrava, Mehran. *The Modern Middle East: A Political History Since the First World War.* Berkeley: University of California Press, 2011.

Khoury, Philip S. *Syria and the French Mandate: the Politics of Arab Nationalism, 1920-1945.* Princeton: Princeton University Press, 1987.

Lane Fox, Robin. *Pagans and Christians.* New York: Alfred A. Knopf, 1987.

Mansfield, Peter. *The Arabs.* New York: Viking Penguin, 1985.

McLaren, Bruce. *The Plain of Dead Cities: A Syrian Tale.* Seattle: Cune Press, 2015.

Moubayed, Sami. *East of the Grand Ummayad: Freemasons in Damascus 1868-1965.* Seattle: Cune Press, 2016.

Moubayed, Sami. *Steel and Silk.* Seattle: Cune Press, 2005.

Muir, William. *The Mameluke. Or Slave Dynasty of Egypt, 1260-1517.* Hong Kong: Forgotten Books, 2012.

al-Nimer, Reem. *The Curse of the Achille Lauro: The Story of Abu al-Abbas.* Seattle: Cune Press, 2014.

Schimmel, Annemarie. *Mystical Dimensions of Islam.* University of North Carolina Press, 1975.

Seale, Patrick. *Asad: The Struggle for the Middle East.* Berkeley: University of California Press, 1989.

Stark, Freya. *The Valleys of the Assassins.* London: John Murray, 1934.

Thomas, Davis, ed. *Syrian Christians Under Islam: The First Thousand Years.* Leiden: Boston: Brill, 2001.

Van Dam, Nikolaos. *The Struggle for Power in Syria: Politics and Society under Asad and the Ba'th Party.* London: I.B. Taurus, 2011.

Wieland, Carsten. *Syria – A Decade of Lost Chances.* Seattle: Cune Press, 2012.

Yazbek, Samar. *A Woman in the Crossfire: Diaries of the Syrian Revolution.* London: Haus Publishing, Ltd, 2012.

Forthcoming books from Cune Press include:

Hamarneh-Hall, Natasha. *Art in Exile: Voices from Yarmouk.* Seattle: Cune Press, 2017.

Hilsman, Patrick. *Gate of Peace, Gate of Wind: Reporting the Syrian Revolution from Behind the Lines.* Seattle: Cune Press, 2017.

Moubayed, Sami. *East of the Grand Umayyad: Freemasons in Syria 1868 - 1965.* Seattle: Cune Press, 2016.

Moubayed, Sami. *Shukri Quwatli: The George Washington of Syria.* Seattle: Cune Press, 2017.

Rifai, Bassam S, *Leaving Syria: Cold, Hunger, Fear—and Humanity.* Seattle: Cune Press, 2016.

Index

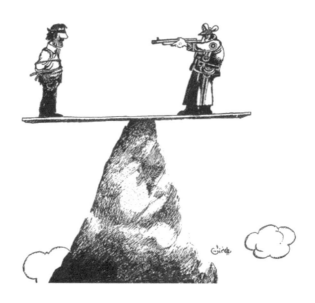

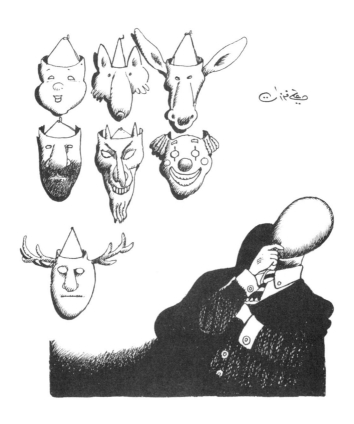

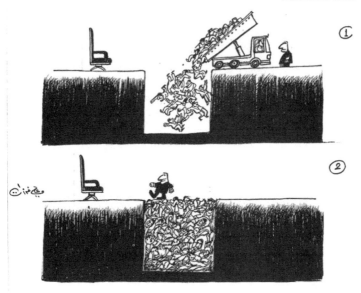

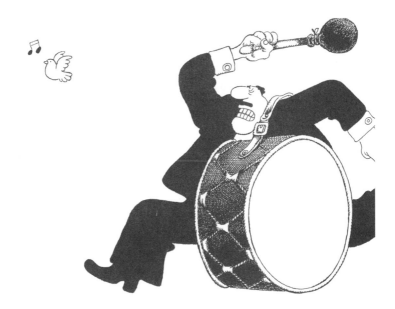

Ali Ferzat

Ali Ferzat (also "Farzat" and "Firzat") is the dean of Syrian political cartoonists. His work has appeared for forty-eight years in major Arab daily newspapers as well as in *Le Monde* and other international publications. Ferzat has served as head of the Society of Arab Cartoonists since 1980 and has won many awards. In October 2011, he and other Arab Spring activists received the Sakharov Rights Prize from the European Parliament. *Time* magazine nominated him as one of the "100 most influential people in the world."

Ferzat was born in the Syrian city of Hama and from his student days lived and worked in Damascus. For years Ferzat published in the Syrian regime's newspaper *Al-Thawra*, where he avoided direct criticism of the president. His favorite targets were the wealthy, the bureaucrats, the military, and the plight of the common man—some of the same themes that Tarif Bakdash sounds in his memoir.

Ferzat was born in 1951, so he is fourteen years older than Tarif Bakdash. In 2001, as Bakdash was preparing to return to Damascus, Ferzat (with the encouragement of the new President Bashar al-Assad) launched his publication *Ad-Domari*—a satirical newspaper that is credited as the first independent publication allowed under Ba'ath rule. It closed under pressure after three years. Tarif Bakdash knew Ferzat personally when he worked for the First Lady's favorite charity AAMAL. Ali Ferzat assisted this group as an illustrator.

With the advent of Arab Spring protests in 2011, Ferzat began to depict the president in his drawings. One caricature showed Bashar Assad standing at the side of a road hitching a ride out of town from Muammar Gaddafi— just before the latter's death. This drawing apparently provoked an attack in August, 2011. Masked men carrying guns kidnapped Ferzat, smashed his fingers to prevent him from continuing his career as a caricaturist, and threw him from a speeding car. Soon after, Ferzat moved to Kuwait.

Ali Ferzat frequently visits Europe and, occasionally, the US. He waits for the time when he can return to his studio on Pakistan Street in Damascus.

For more about Ali Ferzat, see his book or visit him online:
A Pen of Damascus Steel: Political Cartoons of an Arab Master.
For more: www.aliferzat.com

Professor WD Blackmon

Professor WD Blackmon has been the Department Head of the English Department at Missouri State University (a university with 24,000 students) for the past eighteen years. He is the co-founder of the Creative Writing Program in the English Department at Missouri State, a program which has both a strong graduate and undergraduate programs, with the undergraduate program being perhaps the largest such program in the United States (with more than 600 students in the combined programs each semester). As well as doing administrative work, Dr Blackmon also teaches advanced fiction writing in the department.

Professor Blackmon received his PhD at the University of Denver (where he had a teaching fellowship), his Masters of Arts at the University of Utah (where he received a Special Fellowship in the Humanities), and his Bachelors of Arts at the University of Arkansas (where he had an academic scholarship). He also was awarded a full academic scholarship to the University of Texas, but declined that scholarship to attend the University of Arkansas.

Dr Blackmon has won a Book-of-the-Month Club Fellowship Award for his fiction writing (with internationally acclaimed authors Saul Bellow and Ralph Ellison as the judges). He also won the prestigious and competitive Woodrow Wilson Fellowship for university teachers. His short stories have appeared in such publications as the Associated Writing Programs' (organizing the 300 university Creative Writing programs in the United States And Canada) *Intro* series (with RV Cassill as editor), *The Kansas Quarterly*, *The Mississippi Review*, *Short Story*, *The Carolina Quarterly*, and the *Western Humanities Review*. His scholarly writing has appeared most frequently in *The Denver Quarterly*.

Blood and Milk: A Novel in Stories, Professor Blackmon's recent book, was published by Et Alia Press and features photo illustrations from internationally noted photographer Julie Blackmon, whose work has appeared in such publications as *The New Yorker*, *Time* magazine (a cover), Italian *Vogue*, Italian *Vanity Fair*, and *The New York Times Magazine*.
For more: www.wdblackmon.com

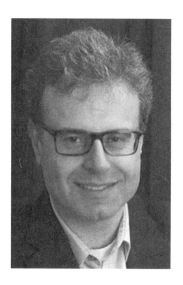

Dr Tarif Bakdash was born in 1965 in Damascus, Syria, graduated from University of Damascus medical school in 1988, and then emigrated to the US. Over the next fourteen years, he held half a dozen positions with institutions as diverse as the Henry Ford Hospital in Detroit and the Harvard Medical School.

In 2002, Dr Bakdash returned to Syria at the invitation of President Bashar al-Assad to teach at the University of Damascus. In addition to his teaching, Dr Bakdash opened a private pediatric neurology clinic. Over the next eight years, he served in Damascus with the World Health Organization of the United Nations. He was named the Services Director and later the National Plan Director for the Syrian Organization for the Disabled (AAMAL) and later was given a government appointment as the first Secretary General for the Disabled in Syria.

In 2010, Dr Bakdash left Syria and returned to the US. He now collaborates with the Syrian American Medical Society (SAMS) on health issues facing Syrian refugees in Jordan and Lebanon. He recently visited the al-Za'atari refugee camp in Jordan to treat Syrian refugees.

In 2015, Dr Bakdash received the Standing Ovation Award from the Children's Hospital of Wisconsin for his humanity in treating children.

For more:
www.bakdash.net
www.cunepress.info/isp